Lecture Notes in Computer Science 16534

The series Lecture Notes in Computer Science (LNCS), including its subseries Lecture Notes in Artificial Intelligence (LNAI) and Lecture Notes in Bioinformatics (LNBI), has established itself as a medium for the publication of new developments in computer science and information technology research, teaching, and education.

LNCS enjoys close cooperation with the computer science R & D community, the series counts many renowned academics among its volume editors and paper authors, and collaborates with prestigious societies. Its mission is to serve this international community by providing an invaluable service, mainly focused on the publication of conference and workshop proceedings and postproceedings. LNCS commenced publication in 1973.

Naren Akash · Cosmin Bercea · Amar Kumar
Editors

Empowering Medical Image Computing and Research Through Early-Career Expertise

Second MICCAI Student Board Workshop, EMERGE 2025
Held in Conjunction with MICCAI 2025
Daejeon, South Korea, September 23, 2025
Proceedings

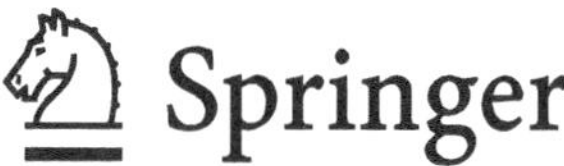

Editors
Naren Akash
IIIT Hyderabad and AIG Hospitals
Hyderabad, Telangana, India

Cosmin Bercea
Technical University of Munich
Munich, Germany

Amar Kumar
McGill University
Montreal, QC, Canada

ISSN 0302-9743 ISSN 1611-3349 (electronic)
Lecture Notes in Computer Science
ISBN 978-3-032-24181-8 ISBN 978-3-032-24182-5 (eBook)
https://doi.org/10.1007/978-3-032-24182-5

This Springer imprint is published by the registered company Springer Nature Switzerland AG
The registered company address is: Gewerbestrasse 11, 6330 Cham, Switzerland

Preface

This volume contains the proceedings of the Second MICCAI Student Board (MSB) Empowering Medical Information Computing and Research Through Early-Career Guidance and Expertise Workshop (MSB EMERGE 2025), held on September 23, 2025, in Daejeon, South Korea, as a half-day satellite event of the 28th International Conference on Medical Image Computing and Computer Assisted Intervention (MICCAI 2025).

EMERGE is a workshop organized by students, for students. It is dedicated to supporting early-career researchers—undergraduate, master's, and doctoral students, as well as recent graduates—in presenting their work, receiving constructive feedback from senior researchers, and developing as independent investigators. The workshop encourages submissions where young scientists are the primary investigators, and in particular where they serve as first or last authors. Oral sessions emphasize mentorship-led discussion over traditional presentation formats to support early-career development.

The first edition of EMERGE was held in 2024 in Marrakesh, Morocco. This second edition built on that foundation with a rigorous review process, a diverse program committee, and a broader scope of accepted contributions. With MICCAI 2025 taking place in South Korea for the first time, this year's program placed particular emphasis on research addressing challenges in the Pan-Asian context, while remaining open to contributions from all regions.

The workshop accepted submissions through two tracks. The Archival Track submissions underwent rigorous double-blind peer review, with each paper evaluated by at least three independent reviewers. The track received 19 submissions, of which 13 were accepted: 9 for oral presentation and 4 conditionally accepted after major revision. All reviews, rebuttals, and preprints of accepted papers are publicly available on the OpenReview platform. Accepted archival papers are published in these Springer LNCS proceedings, and authors of selected papers were invited to submit extended versions to MELBA (The Journal of Machine Learning for Biomedical Imaging). The Non-Archival Track offered authors of accepted MICCAI 2025 main conference posters the opportunity to present their work as oral talks at EMERGE, subject to a light single-blind review for relevance and fit.

The scientific program was organized into three thematic oral sessions: (1) Foundation Models and Generalization in Medical AI, (2) Representation Learning for Detection and Diagnosis, and (3) Signals, Bias, and Structure in Medical Data. A conference-to-workshop track featured flash talks by four MICCAI 2025 poster presenters. The program also included a keynote talk and a poster session with short teasers. The three highest-ranked papers were recognized with awards at the closing ceremony.

The scope of the workshop covered medical image computing and computer-assisted interventions, in line with the scientific goals of the MICCAI Society. Accepted contributions addressed topics including open-set lesion detection, anomaly classification, spectral graph learning, and domain-adaptive contrastive learning. The volume also covers adversarial robustness in segmentation, adaptive watermarking for synthesis, and reinforcement learning for diverse medical image generation.

We thank all authors for their contributions, the program committee members for their thorough and constructive reviews, and the MICCAI 2025 Young Scholars Initiative Committee for their guidance. We also thank the MICCAI 2025 organizers for their logistical support and the MICCAI Student Board for its continued commitment to advancing the scientific and professional development of early-career researchers in our community. The EMERGE initiative is fully supported by the MICCAI Society. This year, the best paper award was sponsored by NVIDIA.

September 2025

Naren Akash
Amar Kumar
Cosmin Bercea

Organization

Organizing Committee and Program Chairs

Naren Akash	IIIT Hyderabad and AIG Hospitals, India
Amar Kumar	McGill University, Canada
Cosmin Bercea	Technical University of Munich, Germany

MICCAI 2025 Young Scholars Initiative Committee

Minjeong Kim	University of North Carolina, USA
Islem Rekik	Imperial College London, UK
Ehsan Adeli	Stanford University, USA
Anees Kazi	Harvard Medical School, USA
Seong Jae Hwang	Yonsei University, South Korea

Program Committee

Amar Kumar	McGill University, Canada
Anees Kazi	Harvard Medical School, USA
Anneliese Riess	Helmholtz Munich, Germany
Cosmin Bercea	Technical University of Munich, Germany
Daniel M. Lang	Helmholtz Munich, Germany
Gurucharan Marthi Krishna Kumar	McGill University, Canada
Johannes Kiechle	Technical University of Munich, Germany
Kumar Abhishek	Simon Fraser University, Canada
Laura Alexandra Daza	Helmholtz Zentrum München, Germany
Lina Felsner	Technical University of Munich, Germany
Marta Hasny	Helmholtz Munich, Germany
Maxime Di Folco	Télécom Paris, France
Moritz Fuchs	Technical University of Darmstadt, Germany
Naren Akash	IIIT Hyderabad and AIG Hospitals, India
Nick Lemke	Technical University of Darmstadt, Germany
Nourhan Bayasi	University of British Columbia, Canada
Sameer Ambekar	Technical University of Munich, Germany
Sushobhan Ghosh	Amazon Research, USA

Contents

Oral Presentations 3: Signals, Bias, and Structure in Medical Data

Poster Presentations

Oral Presentations 1: Foundation Models and Generalization in Medical AI

NFCMTL: Auto NailFold Capillaroscopy Through a Multi-task Learning Model

Yingke Ding[1,3], Jiankai Tang[1], Wanying Mo[1], Tianruo Rose Xu[4], Yuanchun Shi[1,2], and Yuntao Wang[1(✉)]

[1] Tsinghua University, Beijing, China
{dyk21,tjk24,mwy21}@mails.tsinghua.edu.cn,
{shiyc,yuntaowang}@tsinghua.edu.cn
[2] Qinghai University, Qinghai, China
[3] University of Washington, Seattle, WA, USA
[4] Cornell University, Ithaca, NY, USA
tx88@cornell.edu

Abstract. Nailfold capillaroscopy is a non-invasive technique for assessing microvascular health by visualizing capillaries in the nailfold, playing a key role in diagnosing vascular and autoimmune diseases. We propose a novel machine learning approach for nailfold analysis, introducing an advanced multi-task learning model that jointly performs capillary segmentation, classification, and keypoint detection within a unified architecture. Using a large public dataset with reorganized keypoint annotations, our approach improves precision and efficiency in feature detection while simplifying the conventional multi-stage pipeline. By leveraging multi-task optimization, the model achieves state-of-the-art performance comparable to existing methods. This work advances nailfold imaging by providing an accurate, streamlined solution for automated, non-invasive microvascular diagnostics. Code is available at https://github.com/thuhci/NFCMTL.

Keywords: Nailfold Capillaroscopy · Multitask Learning · Vision Transformer

1 Introduction

NailFold Capillaroscopy (NFC) is a non-invasive imaging modality used clinically to assess the health of the microcirculatory system by visualizing capillary structures near the surface of the skin, particularly at the human finger nailfold area [2,4,8]. This imaging technique provides critical insights into capillary morphology, making it indispensable in diagnosing and monitoring a range of autoimmune and vascular conditions, including Systemic Sclerosis (SSc) [13,23] and Raynaud's phenomenon [18,22]. Moreover, emerging research indicates that NFC abnormalities might correlate closely with metabolic disorders such as diabetes [17,24], thus further extending its diagnostic relevance.

N. Akash et al. (Eds.): EMERGE 2025 Workshops, LNCS 16534, pp. 3–12, 2026.
https://doi.org/10.1007/978-3-032-24182-5_1

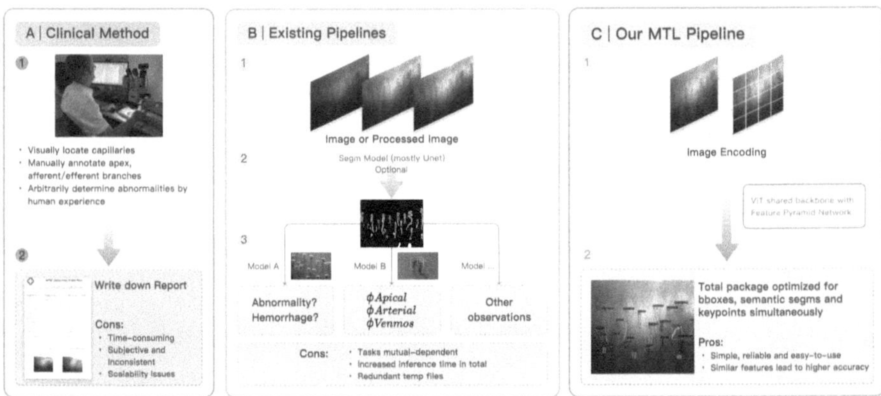

Fig. 1. Traditional method for NFC **(A)** requires significant clinician intervention. While existing deep learning approaches **(B)** allow clinicians to process images through multiple separate models, our proposed multi-task learning model **(C)** integrates key tasks into a unified model that produces comprehensive capillary image analysis in a single operation. Note: the A ① image is obtained from [10].

In traditional clinics, NFC examinations involve capturing microscopic images at approximately $\times 200$ magnification, followed by detailed manual analysis. Specialists visually inspect these images for morphological abnormalities, delineate capillary boundaries, classify capillary morphology, and measure parameters such as apical, arterial, and venous diameters. They then compare these morphological and quantitative findings to reference criteria or rely on clinical experience to identify abnormalities indicative of disease (Fig. 1 **(A)**). While effective, this manual assessment is inherently *subjective, labor-intensive, time-consuming*, and highly *dependent* on clinician expertise, potentially leading to diagnostic variability, inconsistent image interpretation, and delayed or inaccurate clinical decisions [1]. Additionally, the manual approach significantly strains clinical resources, restricting NFC's broader accessibility and clinical adoption.

The application of machine learning in nailfold capillaroscopy is advancing accurate automated diagnosis. A common starting point in this process is segmentation, which outlines targeted capillaries in input images. While not strictly necessary for morphological estimation or parameter calculation, segmentation enhances deep learning pipelines by improving capillary localization [3]. Neural networks like U-Net [21], Mask-RCNN [9] and their variants [16,19] are widely used in NFC segmentation.

Beyond segmentation, capillary classification also plays a crucial role in identifying different capillary types, such as normal, abnormal, or those with conjunctions or anastomoses [7,29]. CNN-based approaches have proven effective for this task. Meanwhile, the quantification of capillary parameters, including density, loop width, and arterial/venous length, is essential for diagnosing diseases like systemic sclerosis, lupus, and rheumatoid arthritis. Some studies favor traditional computer vision or mathematical methods for this analysis [7,12].

Recent viral NFC studies also favor keypoint-based quantitative analysis. For example, Tello et al. [7] employed stacked DenseNet for two-stage capillary parameter estimation, achieving 88% accuracy at a confidence threshold of 0.50. Zhao et al. [29] combined Mask-RCNN with a matching algorithm, reporting an apical diameter MAE of 1.674 pixels and RMSE of 2.023 pixels. Integrating keypoint estimation into NFC analysis enhances accuracy and efficiency.

Despite successes in individual NFC tasks, existing methods fail to **simultaneously** predict multiple tasks. Similar medical imaging studies, such as retinal fundus [28] and skin lesions [25], have demonstrated strong connections between related tasks like classification and segmentation. General imaging applications, including human pose estimation, also indicate a strong link between keypoint estimation and segmentation [6].

To bridge the gap in existing NFC research, we introduce a novel Multi-Task Learning (NFCMTL) strategy, depicted in Fig. 1**(C)**, that integrates capillary *semantic segmentation*, *keypoint detection*, and *classification* into a single unified model. Leveraging a Multiscale Vision Transformer (MViT) backbone with a Feature Pyramid Network (FPN), our model uses a specialized loss function to optimize task predictions simultaneously. Evaluations on the ANFC dataset [29] demonstrate balanced performance improvements across tasks. Ablation studies further confirm precision gains from task unification, achieving sub-pixel accuracy (< 1 pixel error) in downstream capillary parameter estimations.

Our contributions are summarized as follows: **1)** We propose the first reliable multi-task learning model for NFC image tasks, simultaneously performing precise segmentation, classification, and keypoint estimation. **2)** We introduce the **MViT-FPN** model, which outperforms existing approaches in NFC imaging tasks. **3)** Through extensive experiments, NFCMTL demonstrates superior performance in capillary entity estimation and parameter computation, especially when keypoint detection is jointly learned.

2 Method

2.1 Dataset, Annotations, and Keypoints Definition

The dataset comprises N clinician-selected RGB capillaroscopy images of size $W \times H \times 3$, collected from multiple participants. Each image $\mathcal{M}_j$, where $j \in 1, 2, ..., N$, contains several visible capillaries and optional hemorrhages. The capillaries in $\mathcal{M}_j$ are represented as a list of entities $\{\mathcal{E}_1^{(j)}, \mathcal{E}_2^{(j)}, \dots, \mathcal{E}_w^{(j)}\}$, where w is the number of annotated capillaries in $\mathcal{M}_j$.

A capillary entity $\mathcal{E}_i^{(j)}$ can now be written as a tuple of four components:

$$\mathcal{E}_i^{(j)} = \left(\mathcal{S}_i^{(j)}, \mathcal{B}_i^{(j)}, \mathcal{Q}_i^{(j)}, \mathcal{P}_i^{(j)}\right) \tag{1}$$

In Fig. 1, $\mathcal{S}_i^{(j)}$ denotes the segmentation polygon, $\mathcal{B}_i^{(j)}$ refers to the bounding box, $\mathcal{Q}_i^{(j)}$ corresponds to the classification label and $\mathcal{P}_i^{(j)}$ represents the set of keypoints. In this study, we define a fixed set of 9 keypoints, which include the up

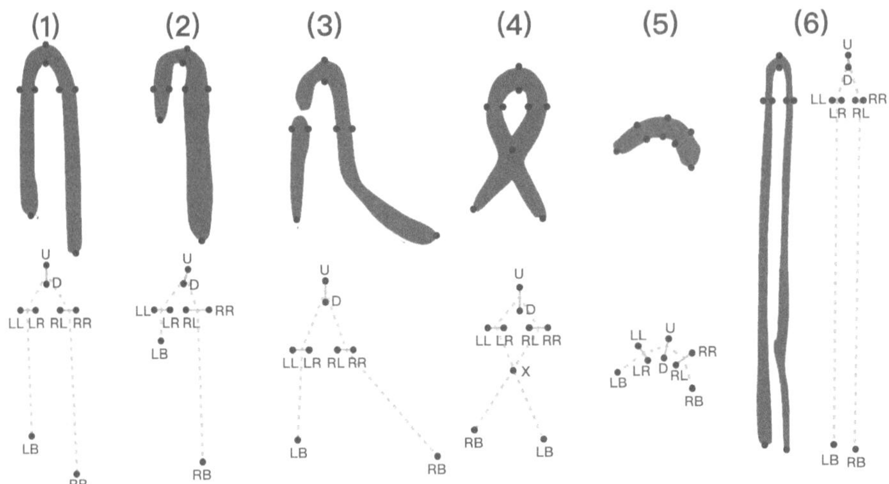

Fig. 2. Different types of nailfold capillaries examined in this research. **(1)** Normal capillary displaying the classic inverted-U shape. **(2)** Abnormal capillary where the afferent limb (left portion) is shorter than the efferent limb (right portion). **(3)** Abnormal capillary characterized by a non-linear efferent limb. **(4)** Abnormal capillary exhibiting a conjunction or anastomosis. **(5)** Abnormal capillary with both afferent and efferent limbs shorter than typical length. **(6)** Abnormal capillary with both afferent and efferent limbs longer than typical length.

(U), down (D), left-left (LL), left-right (LR), right-left (RL), right-right (RR), left-bottom (LB), right-bottom (RB) and the optional conjunction (X). The U and D points are chosen from the capillary apex, LL and LR are selected from the arterial limb, while RL and RR are selected from the venous limb. All keypoints in a capillary entity are represented as one-hot binary masks of size $m \times m$, where each mask encodes a specific anatomical landmark and a spatial softmax over the m^2 grid is applied to predict the most probable keypoint location during inference, as described in [9]. Note that all capillaries in this study must contain the 8 essential keypoints, with the exception of the optional conjunction point. Hemorrhages class do not contain any keypoints. To facilitate better representation of this information, we adopt the MS COCO format [15] for annotations, assigning a visibility flag to each keypoint. Figure 2 illustrates various keypoint annotations in this research.

2.2 Model Architecture

Overview. The architecture of the proposed model is illustrated in Fig. 3. While the final tasks share close relationships, they necessitate distinct prediction strategies due to the intricate characteristics of nailfold capillaries—small size, subtle visual features, occlusions, and irregular shapes. Consequently, the model must effectively capture both low-level visual details and high-level structural relationships. We adopt the Multiscale Vision Transformer (MViT) [5,14] to

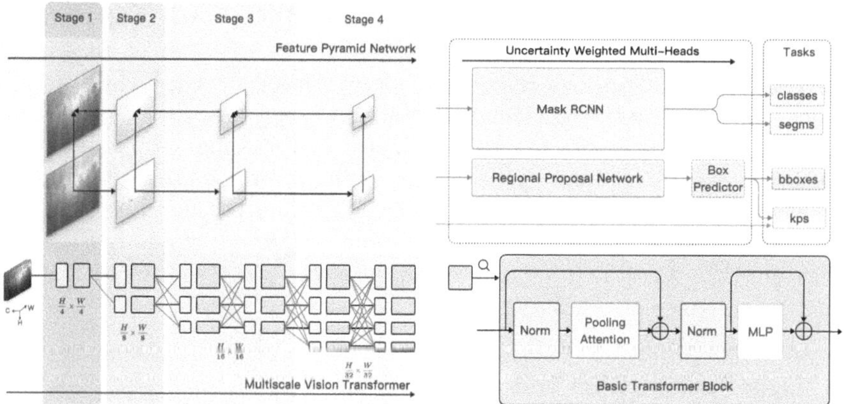

Fig. 3. Overview of the proposed architecture. The model integrates a Multiscale Vision Transformer backbone with a Feature Pyramid Network to capture both fine-grained details and high-level structural context of the capillaries. The multi-scale features are fed into task-specific heads built on Mask R-CNN and Region Proposal Network to perform segmentation masks, classification, and keypoint heatmap tasks.

address these challenges—we encode each input into multi-scale square patches through adaptive upsampling and downsampling operations. These multi-scale patches align naturally with the four-stage Feature Pyramid Network (FPN), subsequently feeding into dedicated task-specific heads—Mask-RCNN [9] and Region Proposal Network (RPN) [20], where a custom total loss function is applied to optimize multi tasks, resulting in a comprehensive prediction of capillary representations.

Backbone. Firstly, all input nailfold capillary images are adopted paddings for a square shape. We then segment the image into $P \times P$ patches. For ViT-based encoding, the model extract features to encode each patch into a multi-scale feature map $\mathbf{F} \in \mathbf{R}^{\frac{H}{P} \times \frac{W}{P} \times D}$. To create multiple feature maps at different scales as used in FPN, we perform recursive down-sampling and up-sampling using convolutional layers with stride $s \sim \{4, 8, 16, 32\}$. Later in the FPN module, we return the feature map to its original resolution by upsampling recursively.

Attention Module. Just like other ViT systems, the attention scores between each pair of patches are computed by taking the dot product between the query Q, key K and value vectors V. Let $X = [x_1, x_2, \ldots, x_N]$ be the sequence of input patch representations, the three vectors can be calculated with learnable weight matrices $Q = XW_Q, K = XW_K, V = XW_V$.

The resulting scores are scaled by $\frac{1}{\sqrt{d}}$, $d = \frac{H}{P} \times \frac{W}{P} \times D$ to stabilize gradients during training. These scores are passed through softmax for weights.

ROI Heads. The downstream ROI heads refine FPN-generated proposals and make final predictions for the capillary tasks with the structure of Mask-RCNN and RPN. The model utilizes ROI Align adopted from the Mask R-CNN framework to extract features from each proposal. Following this, the model performs bounding box regression to adjust coordinates and classifies capillaries using a softmax function. To predict the keypoint heatmap, we use a top-down method that takes the predicted bounding boxes with FPN output features to generate the heatmap. Capillary semantic segmentation is achieved by piping FPN's output features into Mask R-CNN, which then uses five 256×256 Conv2d heads to predict five distinct pixel-level classes.

2.3 Task-Specific Loss and Multitask Loss

Classification Loss. Let $\hat{y}$ be the predicted probability distribution (from the final softmax layer), and y be the true class label (a one-hot encoded vector). The classification loss is hereby $\mathcal{L}_{\text{class}} = -\sum_{c=1}^{C} y_c \log(\hat{y}_c)$, where C is the number of classes, y_c is the true label for class c, and $\hat{y}_c$ is the predicted probability for class c.

Segmentation Loss. We use the *Dice Loss* for segmentation $\mathcal{L}_{\text{segm}} = 1 - \frac{2\sum_i \mathcal{S}_i g_i}{\sum_i \mathcal{S}_i + \sum_i g_i}$. Here $\mathcal{S}_i$ is the predicted segmentation mask at pixel i, and g_i is the ground truth segmentation mask at pixel i.

Bounding Box Loss. For the bounding box regression task, we use the *Smooth L1 Loss*. Let $\mathcal{B}_i^{(j)} = [x_{\text{min}}, y_{\text{min}}, x_{\text{max}}, y_{\text{max}}]$ be the predicted bounding box for the i-th capillary, and $\mathcal{G}_i^{(j)} = [g_{\text{min}}, h_{\text{min}}, g_{\text{max}}, h_{\text{max}}]$ be the ground truth bounding box. The bounding box loss is defined as $\mathcal{L}_{\text{bbox}} = \frac{1}{4}\sum_i \left(\left| \mathcal{B}_i^{(j)} - \mathcal{G}_i^{(j)} \right|^2 \right)$.

Keypoint Loss. For the keypoint detection task, we use the *cross-entropy loss*: $\mathcal{L}_{\text{kp}} = \frac{1}{N}\sum_{n=1}^{N}\sum_{k=1}^{K}\sum_{i=1}^{S}\sum_{j=1}^{S} -g_{n,k,i,j}\log(\hat{g}_{n,k,i,j})$. The predicted keypoints are represented as a tensor of logits of shape (N, K, S, S), where N is the batch size, K is the number of keypoints, and S is the size of the keypoint heatmap. The ground truth keypoints are converted into heatmaps.

Total Loss. Since all tasks here are jointly optimized, weighting strategies are vital for the final optimization. Brought the idea from [11], we use uncertainty weighting to balance these tasks: $\mathcal{L}_{\text{total}} = \mathcal{UW} \otimes \{\mathcal{L}_{\text{class}}, \mathcal{L}_{\text{segm}}, \mathcal{L}_{\text{bbox}}, \mathcal{L}_{\text{kp}}\}$.

Table 1. Summary of evaluation results

Task	Subtask	Metrics	Ours	ANFC [29]	CAPI [7]	Mask-RCNN [9]
Segm.	Capillary Mask	Sens.↑	**0.827**	0.653	—	0.820
KP.	Venous Diameter	MAE↑	1.813	**0.989**	1.274	1.794
KP.	Arterial Diameter	MAE↓	**0.825**	0.849	0.856	1.351
KP.	Apical Diameter	MAE↓	**0.321**	1.674	0.575	1.047
Class.	Abnormal State	Accuracy↑	**0.885**	0.800	0.747	0.839

The test set includes 61 images from various distinct subjects, ensuring no overlap between the subjects in the training and test datasets. Classification metric is calculated per image level and keypoint task's metric is calculated at the pixel level. For the ANFC [29] we report the original results from the paper. For the CAPI [7] and Mask-RCNN [9] results, we implemented the method as described in the original paper and evaluated it on the dataset used in this work.

3 Experiment and Discussion

Dataset. We utilized a public dataset of nailfold videocapillaroscopy images from [29]. This dataset contains 321 high-quality capillaroscopy recordings from 68 participants with a microscope of around ×200 magnification. By submitting Biometrics Dataset Release Agreement, we obtain both the raw image data and its Labelme [26] formatted annotation and converted them to COCO format as described in the above section.

Implementation. Model training was conducted on an NVIDIA GeForce RTX 4090 GPU (24 GB) under Ubuntu 24.04, using Python 3.11.11, PyTorch 2.6.0, and Torchvision 0.21.0. Input images were uniformly resized to 1024 × 1024 and augmented via flipping, cropping, resizing. In addition to those augmentations, we applied photometric transformations like random brightness, contrast, and hue shifts to mimic the highly variable lighting conditions found in outpatient clinics. We select MViTv2-T as the initial checkpoint for its strong performance and lightweight architecture. Optimization employed AdamW with an initial learning rate of 1.6e-4, incorporating linear warm-up and scheduled decay at 52,500, 62,500, and 67,500 iterations. Due to GPU memory constraints, the batch size was fixed at 4. An 80:20 train-test split was applied at the subject level to prevent image overlap across sets. Although it has been suggested that Detectron2 [27] may not be ideal for certain experiments [7], we successfully engineered the core codebase using this platform.

Evaluation Metrics. In this research, different metrics are picked for each task, as shown in Table 1. For each task, we conduct experiments using a five-fold setup and report the aggregated results across the folds.

Table 2. Different task combination and evaluation results

Tasks	Segm (Sens.)	Class (Acc.)	MAE_{apex}	MAE_{venous}	MAE_{arterial}
Segm+Class	0.79	**0.905**	—	—	—
Segm+KP	0.82	—	1.823	2.235	0.942
Class+KP	—	0.819	0.632	2.033	1.725
All tasks	**0.83**	0.885	**0.321**	**1.813**	**0.825**

Results. For segmentation, we evaluate pixel-level sensitivity and obtain an average result of 0.827, outperforming ANFC [29] by demonstrating improved segmentation performance. Regarding CAPI [7], since the original method does not address the segmentation task, we do not include it in this comparison.

For the classification task, we assess results at the *whole-image level.* Our assumption is that if an NFC image contains a single abnormal capillary, the entire image is classified as abnormal. Similarly during evaluation, the inferred classifications of individual capillaries are aggregated to determine the overall image classification. Based on this assumption, we hit an 88.5% accuracy, 89.7% precision, 86.8% recall and 88.2% F1 score.

For the keypoint detection task, we assess model performance through a downstream task: capillary parameter estimation. Specifically, the venous diameter is computed as the Euclidean distance between keypoints LL and LR, the arterial diameter from RL and RR, and the apical diameter from U and D. The mean absolute error (MAE) is calculated as the average difference between the predicted and ground truth diameters for all capillaries at the image level. As shown in Table 1, the model demonstrates strong performance, particularly in estimating arterial and apical diameters.

Ablation Study. Table 2 shows the impact of different task combinations on segmentation, classification, and keypoint performance. The final combined task performs well over major tasks, proving unified optimization works as expected.

4 Conclusion

In this paper we introduce a unified multi-task model for nailfold capillaroscopy that merges segmentation, keypoint detection, and capillary classification. Using a Multiscale vision transformer backbone with Mask R-CNN heads, the model delivers more precise capillary geometry and measurements for capillary parameters. This streamlined approach enhances automated NFC analysis, promising better clinical diagnostics and supporting future multi-task NFC research.

Acknowledgments. This work is supported by the National Key R&D Program of China under Grant No. 2024YFB4505500 & 2024YFB4505503, the National Natural Science Foundation of China under Grant No. 62472244, the Qinghai University Research Ability Enhancement Project (2025KTSA05), the foundation of National

Key Laboratory of Human Factors Engineering under Grant No. HFNKL2024W06, the Tsinghua University Initiative Scientific Research Program, and Undergraduate Education Innovation Grants, Tsinghua University.

Disclosure of Interests. The authors have no competing interests to declare that are relevant to the content of this article.

References

1. Berks, M., et al.: Automated structure and flow measurement—a promising tool in nailfold capillaroscopy. Microvasc. Res. **118**, 173–177 (2018). https://doi.org/10.1016/j.mvr.2018.03.016
2. Berks, M., et al.: An automated system for detecting and measuring nailfold capillaries. In: Golland, P., Hata, N., Barillot, C., Hornegger, J., Howe, R. (eds.) Medical Image Computing and Computer-Assisted Intervention - MICCAI 2014, pp. 658–665. Springer, Cham (2014)
3. Bharathi, P.G., et al.: A deep learning system for quantitative assessment of microvascular abnormalities in nailfold capillary images. Rheumatology **62**(6), 2325–2329 (2023)
4. Etehad Tavakol, M., Fatemi, A., Karbalaie, A., Emrani, Z., Erlandsson, B.E., et al.: Nailfold capillaroscopy in rheumatic diseases: which parameters should be evaluated? BioMed Res. Int. **2015** (2015)
5. Fan, H., et al.: Multiscale vision transformers. In: Proceedings of the IEEE/CVF International Conference on Computer Vision (ICCV), pp. 6824–6835 (2021)
6. Geng, Z., Sun, K., Xiao, B., Zhang, Z., Wang, J.: Bottom-up human pose estimation via disentangled keypoint regression. In: Proceedings of the IEEE/CVF Conference on Computer Vision and Pattern Recognition (CVPR), pp. 14676–14686 (2021)
7. Gracia Tello, B., et al.: The challenge of comprehensive nailfold videocapillaroscopy practice: a further contribution. Clin. Exp. Rheumatol. **40**(10), 1926–1932 (2022). https://doi.org/10.55563/clinexprheumatol/6usce8
8. Hahn, M., Heubach, T., Steins, A., Jünger, M.: Hemodynamics in nailfold capillaries of patients with systemic scleroderma: synchronous measurements of capillary blood pressure and red blood cell velocity. J. Investig. Dermatol. **110**(6), 982–985 (1998)
9. He, K., Gkioxari, G., Dollár, P., Girshick, R.: Mask r-cnn. In: Proceedings of the IEEE International Conference on Computer Vision, pp. 2961–2969 (2017)
10. Jee, A.S., et al.: Nailfold capillaroscopy by smartphone-dermatoscope for connective tissue disease diagnosis in interstitial lung disease: a prospective observational study. ERJ Open Res. **7**(4) (2021). https://doi.org/10.1183/23120541.00416-2021. https://publications.ersnet.org//content/erjor/7/4/00416-2021
11. Kendall, A., Gal, Y., Cipolla, R.: Multi-task learning using uncertainty to weigh losses for scene geometry and semantics. In: Proceedings of the IEEE Conference on Computer Vision and Pattern Recognition (CVPR) (2018)
12. Kim, B., Hariyani, Y.S., Cho, Y.H., Park, C.: Automated white blood cell counting in nailfold capillary using deep learning segmentation and video stabilization. Sensors **20**(24), 7101 (2020)
13. Lambova, S.N., Müller-Ladner, U.: Nailfold capillaroscopy in systemic sclerosis-state of the art: the evolving knowledge about capillaroscopic abnormalities in systemic sclerosis. J. Scleroderma Related Disord. **4**(3), 200–211 (2019)

14. Li, Y., et al.: Mvitv2: improved multiscale vision transformers for classification and detection. In: Proceedings of the IEEE/CVF Conference on Computer Vision and Pattern Recognition (CVPR), pp. 4804–4814 (2022)
15. Lin, T.Y., et al.: Microsoft coco: common objects in context. In: Computer Vision–ECCV 2014: 13th European Conference, Zurich, Switzerland, 6–12 September 2014, Proceedings, Part V 13, pp. 740–755. Springer, Heidelberg (2014)
16. Liu, S., et al.: Segmenting nailfold capillaries using an improved u-net network. Microvasc. Res. **130**, 104011 (2020). https://doi.org/10.1016/j.mvr.2020.104011. https://www.sciencedirect.com/science/article/pii/S0026286220300716
17. Okabe, T., et al.: Relationship between nailfold capillaroscopy parameters and the severity of diabetic retinopathy. Graefes Arch. Clin. Exp. Ophthalmol. **262**(3), 759–768 (2024)
18. Pauling, J.D., Hughes, M., Pope, J.E.: Raynaud's phenomenon—an update on diagnosis, classification and management. Clin. Rheumatol. **38**, 3317–3330 (2019)
19. Qin, X., Zhang, Z., Huang, C., Dehghan, M., Zaiane, O.R., Jagersand, M.: U2-net: going deeper with nested u-structure for salient object detection. Pattern Recogn. **106**, 107404 (2020)
20. Ren, S., He, K., Girshick, R., Sun, J.: Faster r-cnn: towards real-time object detection with region proposal networks. In: Cortes, C., Lawrence, N., Lee, D., Sugiyama, M., Garnett, R. (eds.) Advances in Neural Information Processing Systems, vol. 28. Curran Associates, Inc. (2015). https://proceedings.neurips.cc/paper_files/paper/2015/file/14bfa6bb14875e45bba028a21ed38046-Paper.pdf
21. Ronneberger, O., Fischer, P., Brox, T.: U-net: convolutional networks for biomedical image segmentation. In: International Conference on Medical Image Computing and Computer-Assisted Intervention, pp. 234–241. Springer, Heidelberg (2015)
22. Ruaro, B., et al.: Innovations in the assessment of primary and secondary Raynaud's phenomenon. Front. Pharmacol. **10**, 360 (2019)
23. Ruaro, B., et al.: Advances in nailfold capillaroscopic analysis in systemic sclerosis. J. Scleroderma Related Disord. **3**(2), 122–131 (2018)
24. Shah, R., et al.: Nailfold capillaroscopy and deep learning in diabetes. J. Diabetes **15**(2), 145–151 (2023)
25. Thwin, S.M., Park, H.S.: Enhanced skin lesion segmentation and classification through ensemble models. Eng **5**(4), 2805–2820 (2024)
26. Wada, K.: Labelme: Image polygonal annotation with python (2021). https://doi.org/10.5281/zenodo.5711226. https://github.com/wkentaro/labelme, version as cited on Zenodo. Licensed under GPL-3.0. ORCID: 0000-0002-6347-5156
27. Wu, Y., Kirillov, A., Massa, F., Lo, W.Y., Girshick, R.: Detectron2 (2019). https://github.com/facebookresearch/detectron2
28. Yi, J., Chen, C.: Multi-task segmentation and classification network for artery/vein classification in retina fundus. Entropy **25**(8), 1148 (2023)
29. Zhao, L., et al.: A comprehensive dataset and automated pipeline for nailfold capillary analysis. In: 2024 IEEE International Symposium on Biomedical Imaging (ISBI), pp. 1–5. IEEE (2024)

Foundation Models as Class-Incremental Learners for Dermatological Image Classification

Mohamed Elkhayat[1], Mohamed Mahmoud[1], Jamil Fayyad[2], and Nourhan Bayasi[3(✉)]

[1] Cairo University, Giza, Egypt
{Mohammed.Khayyat02,muhammad.mahmoud01}@eng-st.cu.edu.eg
[2] University of Victoria, Victoria, BC, Canada
[3] University of British Columbia, Vancouver, BC, Canada
nourhanbayasi92@gmail.com

Abstract. Class-Incremental Learning (CIL) aims to learn new classes over time without forgetting previously acquired knowledge. The emergence of foundation models (FM) pretrained on large datasets presents new opportunities for CIL by offering rich, transferable representations. However, their potential for enabling incremental learning in dermatology remains largely unexplored. In this paper, we systematically evaluate frozen FMs pretrained on large-scale skin lesion datasets for CIL in dermatological disease classification. We propose a simple yet effective approach where the backbone remains frozen, and a lightweight MLP is trained incrementally for each task. This setup achieves state-of-the-art performance without forgetting, outperforming regularization, replay, and architecture-based methods. To further explore the capabilities of frozen FMs, we examine zero-training scenarios using nearest-mean classifiers with prototypes derived from their embeddings. Through extensive ablation studies, we demonstrate that this prototype-based variant can also achieve competitive results. Our findings highlight the strength of frozen FMs for continual learning in dermatology and support their broader adoption in real-world medical applications. Our code and datasets are available here.

Keywords: Class-Incremental Learning · Continual Learning · Foundation Models · Dermatological Image Classification · Dermatology

1 Introduction

Real-world clinical applications rarely offer the luxury of independent and identically distributed (i.i.d.) data [15]. In dermatology, new disease classes or imaging variations may appear gradually as data is collected over time from different

M. Elkhayat and M. Mahmoud—Equal contribution.
J. Fayyad and N. Bayasi—Equal engineering contribution.

N. Akash et al. (Eds.): EMERGE 2025 Workshops, LNCS 16534, pp. 13–23, 2026.
https://doi.org/10.1007/978-3-032-24182-5_2

sources. Conventional models trained in a static setting often fail under these changing conditions [16], showing a sharp drop in performance on previously learned tasks when updated with new data; a problem known as *catastrophic forgetting* [4,26]. Continual learning (CL) aims to address this challenge by allowing models to learn new information while preserving past knowledge. Several setups within CL include Class-Incremental Learning (CIL) is one of the most challenging. In CIL, new classes are introduced over time, and the model must learn them without access to data from earlier tasks, making this a relevant setting in clinical workflows where storing or replaying patient data is often restricted due to privacy and ethical concerns.

To avoid forgetting without storing or replaying old patient data [11], researchers have explored regularization- and architecture-based strategies. Regularization methods penalize changes to important parameters [32], while architecture-based approaches expand the model or allocate task-specific components [5,10,36]. While effective in controlled settings, these methods face key limitations in clinical practice: regularization requires reliable importance estimates, which are often difficult to obtain in data-scarce environments, and architecture-based techniques introduce complexity and memory overhead. In contrast, foundation models (FM) trained on large-scale datasets have reshaped the landscape of CIL, offering robust, transferable features that generalize well with minimal fine-tuning [12]. Recent work in natural image domains shows that simply leveraging frozen FMs can significantly boost performance and reduce forgetting [19,20].

Motivated by these findings, we turn to dermatology and ask: Can frozen FMs pretrained on large-scale dermatological data support CIL for skin lesion classification, or are specialized CL methods still necessary? To answer this, we present the first comprehensive evaluation of frozen dermatology FMs for continual skin lesion classification. Our setup is deliberately simple: the backbone remains frozen, and a lightweight MLP classifier is incrementally trained for each task. Surprisingly, this approach outperforms prior CIL methods, including regularization, replay, and architectural techniques, without requiring any fine-tuning. We also explore zero-training setups using prototype-based classifiers derived from FM embeddings, and through extensive ablation studies, demonstrate that variations of this method can significantly outperform existing approaches. Our results suggest that future dermatology-based CL research should start with FMs, rather than designing methods from scratch.

2 Related Work

Class-Incremental Learning for Medical Imaging. CIL has recently received growing attention in medical imaging, driven by the need for models that can learn new disease categories without forgetting prior knowledge, all while preserving patient privacy. This has spurred data-free methods that synthesize prior class representations instead of storing raw images. For example, Ayromlou et al. [1] use gradient inversion and novel loss functions to preserve class discriminability. Bayasi et al. [6,7,9] introduce a pruning-based approach that builds independent subnetworks to eliminate forgetting and support fair and generalizable CL. Others rely on regularization: Chee et al. [13] expand network capacity while retaining prior knowledge, and Chen et al. [14] use contrastive learning and distillation for class- and domain-incremental segmentation.

Foundation Models in Continual Learning. Traditional CL methods often train feature extractors from scratch, making them vulnerable to catastrophic forgetting. Recent work has shown that leveraging frozen FMs can improve both stability and efficiency. In vision, methods like DualPrompt [30] and L2P [31] use prompt tuning on frozen backbones, while Janson et al. [19] showed that simple classifiers on frozen features can rival or outperform complex methods. In medical imaging, Yang et al. [34] used fixed encoders with Gaussian mixtures, Zhang et al. [35] introduced adapter modules, and Bayasi et al. [8] leveraged frozen model ensembles. Yet, the role of FMs in continual dermatology classification remains unexplored, leaving an important gap in the field.

3 Methodology

3.1 Problem Setup

Let $\mathcal{D} = \{(\mathbf{x}_i, y_i)\}_{i=1}^{N}$ denote a dataset of skin lesion images, where $\mathbf{x}_i \in \mathbb{R}^{H\times W\times C}$ is an input image and $y_i \in \{1, 2, \ldots, C\}$ is its corresponding class label. In the class-incremental learning (CIL) setup, the complete set of classes $\mathcal{C} = \{1, 2, ..., C\}$ is partitioned into T disjoint subsets, $\mathcal{C}_1, \mathcal{C}_2, ..., \mathcal{C}_T$, such that new classes are introduced sequentially over T tasks. At each time step $t \in \{1, \ldots, T\}$, the model receives access only to a task-specific dataset $\mathcal{D}_t = \{(\mathbf{x}_i, y_i) \mid y_i \in \mathcal{C}_t\}$. No access is granted to prior task data $\mathcal{D}_{<t}$, and storage of past examples is not allowed. The model must update its classification capabilities to accommodate new classes in $\mathcal{C}_t$ while preserving performance on all previously learned classes $\mathcal{C}_{<t} = \bigcup_{j=1}^{t-1} \mathcal{C}_j$.

Let $\mathcal{F}_\theta$ be a dermatology FM with frozen parameters θ, pretrained on a large-scale skin lesion images. The parameters θ remain fixed and are never updated during the continual learning (CL) process. For an input image $\mathbf{x}$, the model produces a feature embedding:

$$\mathbf{z} = \mathcal{F}_\theta(\mathbf{x}) \in \mathbb{R}^d \quad .$$

Our goal is to evaluate two CL baselines built on top of these frozen embeddings. The first one uses an MLP-based classifier, where a lightweight multi-layer perceptron is incrementally trained on top of the frozen embeddings for each new task. The second one adopts a prototype-based nearest-mean classifier (NMC), which requires no training. Instead, it computes a mean feature vector (prototype) for each class using the frozen features of the labeled training samples.

3.2 Baseline 1: MLP-Based Class-Incremental Learning

In this baseline, we keep the FM frozen and train a lightweight MLP classifier incrementally across tasks.

3.2.1 Training Phase At each task t, a new MLP head $h_t : \mathbb{R}^d \rightarrow \mathbb{R}^{|\mathcal{C}_t|}$ is trained on the frozen embeddings from $\mathcal{D}_t$. The MLP has two hidden layers with ReLU activation and a softmax output:

$$h_t(\mathbf{z}) = \text{Softmax}\left(W_3 \cdot \text{ReLU}\left(W_2 \cdot \text{ReLU}(W_1\mathbf{z} + \mathbf{b}_1) + \mathbf{b}_2\right) + \mathbf{b}_3\right) \ .$$

To support all seen classes, we concatenate the outputs of all MLPs learned up to task t: $h(\mathbf{z}) = \text{Concat}(h_1(\mathbf{z}), \dots, h_t(\mathbf{z}))$.

3.2.2 Inference Phase At test time, input image $\mathbf{x}$ is passed through the frozen encoder and all MLP heads. The final prediction is made by taking the class with the highest probability across all tasks: $\hat{y} = \arg\max_{c \in \mathcal{C}_{\leq t}} h(\mathcal{F}_\theta(\mathbf{x}))_c$.

3.3 Baseline 2: Prototype-Based Nearest Mean Classifier (NMC)

This baseline avoids training by using class-wise mean embeddings (prototypes) computed from frozen features.

3.3.1 Training Phase For each class $c \in \mathcal{C}_t$, we compute a class prototype μ_c by averaging the frozen embeddings of all class-wise training samples in $\mathcal{D}_t$:

$$\mu_c = \frac{1}{|\mathcal{D}_c|} \sum_{(\mathbf{x}_i, y_i) \in \mathcal{D}_t, y_i = c} \mathcal{F}_\theta(\mathbf{x}_i) \ .$$

These prototypes are stored in a memory bank: $\mathcal{M}_t = \{\mu_c \mid c \in \mathcal{C}_t\}$.

3.3.2 Inference Phase Given a test image $\mathbf{x}$, we extract its embedding $\mathbf{z} = \mathcal{F}_\theta(\mathbf{x})$, then classify it by assigning the label of the nearest prototype across all seen classes: $\hat{y} = \arg\min_{c \in \mathcal{C}_{\leq t}} \|\mathbf{z} - \mu_c\|_2$.

4 Experiments and Results

We evaluate our two `FM`-based `CL` baselines on the task of skin lesion classification under the `CIL` setting, where new sets of classes are introduced sequentially without access to previous data. Details are given next.

4.1 Experimental Setup

Datasets. Our experiments are conducted on three publicly available dermatology datasets: HAM10000 (HAM) [28], Dermofit (DMF) [2], and Derm7pt (D7P) [21], comprising 10,015 1,211, and 963 dermoscopic images, respectively. These datasets were collected from diverse clinical sources and span a subset of seven skin lesion classes. To simulate a `CIL` scenario, each dataset is partitioned into T tasks with mutually exclusive class labels. We adopt the dataset splits and experimental protocol from [8] to ensure fair and consistent comparison.

Implementation Details. We evaluate our baselines using two dermatology-based FMs: the Google Derm model [18], a publicly released FM trained on over 400 skin conditions, and PanDerm [33], a large-scale FM pre-trained on millions of clinical and dermoscopic dermatology images. Both models are used as frozen feature extractors throughout the continual learning process, with no fine-tuning. The MLP-based classifier is trained using the Adam optimizer (learning rate 0.001, batch size 200) with cross-entropy loss. Training runs for up to 200 epochs per task, with early stopping based on validation accuracy to mitigate overfitting.

Reference Methods and Competitors. We compare our baselines with three standard reference methods: SINGLE, which trains separate models for different tasks and deploys a specific model for each task during inference; JOINT, which aggregates the data from all tasks as a consolidated dataset to jointly train a single model (aka. multitask learning); and SeqFT, which fine-tunes a single model on the current task, without any countermeasure to forgetting. We compare against several CL competitors, including two regularization-based methods: EWC [22] and LwF [23]; two generative-based method: DGM [25] and BIR [29]; two replay-based method: iCaRL [27] and RM [3] and a frozen pre-trained model-based method: Continual-Zoo [8].

Evaluation Metrics. We report the balanced accuracy (**BAAC**), which accounts for class imbalance by averaging the recall across all classes, ensuring that each class contributes equally to the final score. Also, we report the forgetting measure (**F**), which quantifies how much the model forgets previously learned tasks: $\mathbf{F} = \frac{1}{T-1} \sum_{i=1}^{T-1} \max_{k \in \{1,\dots,T-1\}} a_{k,i} - a_{T,i}$, where $a_{k,i}$ is the accuracy on task i after training on task k, and $a_{T,i}$ is the final accuracy on task i after training on all T tasks. A higher value of **F** indicates more forgetting.

4.2 Results and Analysis

Main Results. Table 1 summarizes the performance of our two FM-based baselines across three skin lesion benchmarks. Our MLP-based models (Google Derm and PanDerm) consistently achieve state-of-the-art balanced accuracy (BAAC) while exhibiting zero forgetting ($\mathbf{F} = 0$), outperforming all existing CL methods including regularization, replay, and architecture-based approaches. On the HAM dataset, PanDerm with MLP achieves a BAAC of 92.25%, surpassing even the upper-bound SINGLE model (88.35%) and strongly outperforming replay-based methods like RM. Similar trends are observed on DMF, where PanDerm with MLP reaches 93.11%, exceeding the best non-foundation continual learning method, Continual-Zoo, by over 20% points. On the D7P dataset, PanDerm again leads with a BAAC of 77.80%, outperforming all methods.

Interestingly, our NMC-based FM baselines, particularly with Google Derm, achieve comparable, and sometimes superior, results relative to other competing techniques. For example, NMC with Google Derm on D7P surpasses all CL methods and even JOINT. However, their performance lag behind their MLP counterparts, reflecting their inability to adapt to complex or overlapping class boundaries typical of medical imaging and skin lesion data. By contrast, MLPs can learn more flexible decision boundaries in the embedding space, better leveraging the rich features of the frozen FM. These results suggest that the choice of classifier plays an important role in realizing the full potential of frozen foundation features in the CIL setting. Motivated by this, we explore enhancements for NMC-based models in the subsequent ablation studies.

Table 1. Performance evaluation of our FM-based baselines and existing methods on three skin lesion classification benchmarks in the CIL setting. Numbers in parentheses next to replay- or generative-based methods indicate the number of stored or generated samples per old class, respectively. [illegible] and blue cells denote the best and second-best results, respectively.

Method	HAM		DMF		D7P	
	BAAC (↑)	**F (↓)**	**BAAC (↑)**	**F (↓)**	**BAAC (↑)**	**F (↓)**
Reference Methods						
SINGLE	88.35	-	85.01	-	73.74	-
JOINT	82.13	-	80.66	-	68.32	-
SeqFT	51.54	50.76	37.21	55.25	36.51	52.18
Competing Methods						
EWC	59.84	32.29	50.86	43.72	42.73	38.51
LWF	61.22	33.70	49.87	40.69	40.67	35.66
DGM	75.97	19.27	64.99	25.47	61.24	22.38
BIR	74.39	17.85	61.47	19.18	62.90	19.65
iCaRL (50)	70.80	18.44	64.32	20.17	60.84	24.78
iCaRL (100)	73.27	14.97	68.49	18.27	63.72	19.28
RM (50)	73.61	16.83	63.73	16.73	63.05	22.57
RM (100)	76.32	15.92	70.14	15.22	65.87	20.17
Continual-Zoo	78.15	11.09	72.51	14.21	68.04	17.58
Ours (Baseline 1: FM with MLP)						
Google Derm	89.26	0	91.35	0	74.59	0
PanDerm	**92.25**	0	**93.11**	0	**77.80**	0
Ours (Baseline 2: FM with NMC)						
Google Derm	64.75	0	67.56	0	68.74	0
PanDerm	57.95	0	49.27	0	44.51	0

Ablation Studies. We conduct ablation studies to understand design choices in our approach: (1) exploring variants of the NMC classifier, and (2) evaluating the impact of replacing dermatology-specific FMs with general-purpose alternatives.

1. NMC Classifier Variants. Table 2 reports the performance of several variants of the base NMC evaluated on HAM, DMF and D7P benchmarks. We begin with a straightforward yet effective enhancement: applying ℓ_2 normalization to embeddings prior to centroid computation. This standardization consistently improves accuracy by better aligning the embedding space for distance-based decisions. For example, on DMF with Google Derm, accuracy increases from 67.56% to 69.46%. Next, we explore projection-based variants that transform embeddings before classification. Random projection [24] into a higher-dimensional Euclidean space yields limited gains; however, when combined with normalization, modest improvements are observed; for instance, PanDerm accuracy on DMF increases from 49.57% to 54.38%. The most substantial improvements arise from our learnable hyperbolic projection [17], which maps embeddings onto a hyperbolic manifold whose parameters are optimized during training. This projection explicitly captures hierarchical and relational structures among classes, adapting the embedding geometry to improve clustering and distance-based decision boundaries. The impact is significant: on HAM, accuracy rises from 64.75% to 81.41% with the Google Derm model and from 57.95% to 80.24% with PanDerm. Further, combining the hyperbolic projection with normalization boosts PanDerm accuracy on D7P from 44.51% to 63.73%, yielding the strongest NMC results overall. While both the hyperbolic projection and the MLP classifier involve learnable parameters, they differ fundamentally. The MLP learns flexible, general mappings from embeddings to class predictions, requiring more extensive training. In contrast, the hyperbolic projection embeds data in a geometric space that models hierarchies, enhancing clustering and interpretability with fewer parameters and less risk of overfitting. We finally assess classical dimensionality reduction techniques. Principal component analysis (PCA), which preserves variance without explicitly optimizing class separability, does not improve performance, whereas Linear discriminant analysis (LDA), designed to maximize between-class variance, delivers mixed, unstable results: while it achieves 78.91% on HAM with PanDerm, its performance deteriorates on other datasets due to the high intra-class variance. In summary, we conclude that normalization (as a non-learnable enhancement) and the hyperbolic projection (as a learnable enhancement) provide the most effective improvements to the NMC, each helping to narrow the gap to the MLP classifiers reported in Table 1 on different datasets.

2. General-Purpose vs. Domain-Specific `FMs`. To assess the importance of domain specialization, we repeat our experiments using a general-purpose `FM`–CLIP ViT-L/14 pretrained on natural images, replacing the dermatology-specific model. Results are shown in Table 3. Despite lacking domain-specific pretraining, CLIP embeddings remain highly effective for parametric classifiers: the MLP achieves 88.38%, 90.43%, and 71.19% on HAM, DMF, and D7P, respectively, outperforming all prior `CL` methods. This supports our central claim: strong, transferable `FM` features, regardless of domain, can improve performance in `CIL`. In contrast, NMC variants suffer significant degradation. The base NMC achieves only 53.53% on HAM and 46.01% on D7P, far below its dermatology-initialized

Table 2. Performance evaluation (balanced accuracy %) of different variations of the NMC classifier across three skin lesion classification benchmarks. cells denote the best results.

Method	HAM		DMF		D7P	
	Derm	PanDerm	Derm	PanDerm	Derm	PanDerm
Base NMC (from Table 1)	64.75	57.95	67.56	49.27	**68.74**	44.51
Base NMC + Norm.	66.60	61.03	**69.46**	**54.89**	66.43	47.94
Random Projection	67.29	57.43	66.99	49.57	68.74	40.72
Random Projection + Norm.	66.11	62.06	66.20	54.38	68.46	47.27
Hyperbolic Projection	**81.41**	**80.24**	63.79	43.21	65.28	59.59
Hyperbolic Projection + Norm.	80.15	80.15	60.08	53.91	64.77	**63.73**
PCA	64.75	56.67	67.26	50.23	68.74	44.51
PCA + Norm.	66.60	59.96	69.46	54.89	66.10	47.94
LDA	51.88	78.91	69.38	37.12	45.23	38.56

Table 3. Performance evaluation (balanced accuracy %) of our FM-based baselines using a general-purpose foundation model (CLIP ViT-L/14). and blue cells denote the best and second-best results, respectively.

Method	HAM	DMF	D7P
Our Baselines			
FM with MLP	**88.38**	**90.43**	**71.19**
FM with NMC	53.53	70.13	46.01
NMC Classifier Variants			
Base NMC + Norm.	55.11	71.26	46.52
Random Projection	52.15	69.99	43.79
Random Projection + Norm.	51.56	69.87	43.63
Hyperbolic Projection	80.05	53.50	59.59
Hyperbolic Projection + Norm.	80.05	57.20	60.10
PCA	53.53	70.13	45.86
PCA + Norm.	55.10	71.25	46.37
LDA	73.04	61.82	28.57

counterpart. Interestingly, while normalization and hyperbolic projection again improve performance (e.g., HAM jumps from 53.53% to 80.05%), they cannot fully bridge the gap, and their gains are inconsistent across datasets. Hyperbolic projection + normalization achieves a strong 60.10% on D7P but still trails the MLP by more than 11%. LDA continues to show erratic behavior: while it produces 73.04% on HAM (competitive with more structured NMC variants), it collapses entirely on D7P (28.57%), underscoring its sensitivity to class imbalance and feature distributions. Overall, these findings reinforce two observations: (1) parametric models like MLPs can extract meaningful decision boundaries from general-purpose FMs, making them highly effective for CIL; and (2) for other approaches like NMC that lack task-specific adaptation, alignment between the pretraining and target domain remains crucial.

5 Conclusions

This work demonstrates the clear advantage of leveraging frozen foundation models as class-incremental learners in dermatological image classification. Through systematic evaluation across three skin lesion benchmarks, we show that a simple approach, which is training a lightweight MLP on top of a frozen dermatology-specific backbone, can surpass upper-bound reference methods, without requiring complex regularization, replay, or architectural modifications. Remarkably, this MLP-based strategy maintains strong performance when built on general-purpose models like CLIP ViT-L/14, further reinforcing the value of rich, pretrained features in CL for medical applications. These findings yield three key insights. First, foundation models should be considered the default starting point for future research in CL. Second, nearest-mean classifiers still benefit substantially from domain-specific pretraining due to their limited representational flexibility. Third, our results emphasize the importance of aligning model design with the geometric properties of the embedding space. Specifically, incorporating inductive biases, such as learnable hyperbolic projections, can significantly close the gap between simple prototype-based classifiers and other learnable models while offering greater simplicity and interpretability. Taken together, we hope this work encourages the community to rethink the foundations of CL; i.e., shifting from building methods from scratch toward designing smarter, lighter learning systems that build on the strengths of powerful pretrained models. A promising future direction is to explore dynamic backbone adaptation and task-aware prompt tuning to further improve flexibility while retaining the benefits of strong pretrained representations.

References

1. Ayromlou, S., Tsang, T., Abolmaesumi, P., Li, X.: CCSI: continual class-specific impression for data-free class incremental learning. Med. Image Anal. (2024)
2. Ballerini, L., Fisher, R.B., Aldridge, B., Rees, J.: A color and texture based hierarchical k-nn approach to the classification of non-melanoma skin lesions. In: Color Medical Image Analysis, pp. 63–86. Springer, Heidelberg (2013)
3. Bang, J., Kim, H., Yoo, Y., Ha, J.W., Choi, J.: Rainbow memory: continual learning with a memory of diverse samples. In: IEEE/CVF CVPR, pp. 8218–8227 (2021)
4. Bayasi, N.: Beyond catastrophic forgetting: advancing continual learning for robust and fair medical image analysis. Ph.D. thesis, University of British Columbia (2025)
5. Bayasi, N., Du, S., Hamarneh, G., Garbi, R.: Continual-gen: continual group ensembling for domain-agnostic skin lesion classification. In: International Conference on Medical Image Computing and Computer-Assisted Intervention (MICCAI), pp. 3–13 (2023)

6. Bayasi, N., Fayyad, J., Bissoto, A., Hamarneh, G., Garbi, R.: Biaspruner: debiased continual learning for medical image classification. In: International Conference on Medical Image Computing and Computer-Assisted Intervention (MICCAI), pp. 90–101. Springer, Heidelberg (2024)
7. Bayasi, N., Hamarneh, G., Garbi, R.: Culprit-prune-net: efficient continual sequential multi-domain learning with application to skin lesion classification. In: International Conference on Medical Image Computing and Computer-Assisted Intervention (MICCAI), pp. 165–175. Springer, Heidelberg (2021)
8. Bayasi, N., Hamarneh, G., Garbi, R.: Continual-zoo: leveraging zoo models for continual classification of medical images. In: Proceedings of the IEEE/CVF Conference on Computer Vision and Pattern Recognition, pp. 4128–4138 (2024)
9. Bayasi, N., Hamarneh, G., Garbi, R.: GC^2: generalizable continual classification of medical images. IEEE Trans. Med. Imaging (2024)
10. Bayasi, N., Saleh, H., Mohammad, B., Ismail, M.: The revolution of glucose monitoring methods and systems: a survey. In: 2013 IEEE 20th International Conference on Electronics, Circuits, and Systems (ICECS), pp. 92–93 (2013)
11. Bera, S., Ummadi, V., Sen, D., Mandal, S., Biswas, P.K.: Memory replay for continual medical image segmentation through atypical sample selection. In: MICCAI, pp. 513–522 (2023)
12. Bommasani, R., et al.: On the opportunities and risks of foundation models. arXiv preprint arXiv:2108.07258 (2021)
13. Chee, E., Lee, M.L., Hsu, W.: Leveraging old knowledge to continually learn new classes in medical images. In: Proceedings of the AAAI Conference on Artificial Intelligence, vol. 37, pp. 14178–14186 (2023)
14. Chen, X., Zheng, H., Xie, Y., Ma, Y., Li, T.: A classifier-free incremental learning framework for scalable medical image segmentation. arXiv preprint arXiv:2405.16328 (2024)
15. Fayyad, J.: Out-of-distribution detection using inter-level features of deep neural networks. Ph.D. thesis, University of British Columbia (2023)
16. Fayyad, J., Alijani, S., Najjaran, H.: Empirical validation of conformal prediction for trustworthy skin lesions classification. Comput. Methods Programs Biomed. **253**, 108231 (2024)
17. Gonzalez-Jimenez, A., et al.: Is hyperbolic space all you need for medical anomaly detection? (2025). Provisionally accepted at MICCAI 2025
18. Google Health AI: Derm foundation model (2025). https://developers.google.com/health-ai-developer-foundations/derm-foundation
19. Janson, P., Zhang, W., Aljundi, R., Elhoseiny, M.: A simple baseline that questions the use of pretrained models in continual learning. In: NeurIPS (2023)
20. Javed, K., Wang, Y., Xu, Q., Zhang, Y.: Parametric prompt tuning for vision-language models. In: CVPR (2023)
21. Kawahara, J., Daneshvar, S., Argenziano, G., Hamarneh, G.: Seven-point checklist and skin lesion classification using multitask multimodal neural nets. IEEE J. Biomed. Health Inf. **23**(2), 538–546 (2018)
22. Kirkpatrick, J., et al.: Overcoming catastrophic forgetting in neural networks. Proc. Natl. Acad. Sci. **114**(13), 3521–3526 (2017)
23. Li, Z., Hoiem, D.: Learning without forgetting. IEEE Trans. Pattern Anal. Mach. Intell. **40**(12), 2935–2947 (2017)
24. McDonnell, M.D., Gong, D., Parveneh, A., Abbasnejad, E., van den Hengel, A.: Ranpac: random projections and pre-trained models for continual learning. arXiv preprint arXiv:2307.02251 (2023). https://doi.org/10.48550/arXiv.2307.02251

25. Ostapenko, O., Puscas, M., Klein, T., Jahnichen, P., Nabi, M.: Learning to remember: a synaptic plasticity driven framework for continual learning. In: CVPR, pp. 11321–11329 (2019)
26. Ratcliff, R.: Connectionist models of recognition memory: constraints imposed by learning and forgetting functions. Psychol. Rev. **97**(2), 285 (1990)
27. Rebuffi, S.A., Kolesnikov, A., Sperl, G., Lampert, C.H.: iCaRL: incremental classifier and representation learning. In: IEEE/CVF CVPR, pp. 2001–2010 (2017)
28. Tschandl, P., Rosendahl, C., Kittler, H.: The HAM10000 dataset, a large collection of multi-source dermatoscopic images of common pigmented skin lesions. Sci. Data **5**(1), 1–9 (2018)
29. van de Ven, G.M., Siegelmann, H.T., Tolias, A.S.: Brain-inspired replay for continual learning with artificial neural networks. Nat. Commun. **11**(1), 1–14 (2020)
30. Wang, Z., et al.: Dualprompt: complementary prompting for rehearsal-free continual learning. In: ECCV, pp. 631–648 (2022)
31. Wang, Z., et al.: Learning to prompt for continual learning. In: IEEE/CVF CVPR, pp. 139–149 (2022)
32. Wu, Z., Zhu, F., Guo, K., Sheng, R., Chao, L., Fang, H.: Modal adaptive super-resolution for medical images via continual learning. Signal Process. (2024)
33. Yan, S., et al.: A general-purpose multimodal foundation model for dermatology. arXiv preprint arXiv:2410.15038 (2024)
34. Yang, Y., Cui, Z., Xu, J., Zhong, C., Zheng, W.S., Wang, R.: Continual learning with bayesian model based on a fixed pre-trained feature extractor. Visual Intell. **1**(1), 5 (2023)
35. Zhang, W., Huang, Y., Zhang, T., Zou, Q., Zheng, W.S., Wang, R.: Adapter learning in pretrained feature extractor for continual learning of diseases. In: MICCAI, pp. 68–78 (2023)
36. Zhang, Y., Li, X., Chen, H., Yuille, A.L., Liu, Y., Zhou, Z.: Continual learning for abdominal multi-organ and tumor segmentation. In: MICCAI (2023)

ZeroSlide: Is Zero-Shot Classification Adequate for Lifelong Learning in Whole-Slide Image Analysis in the Era of Pathology Vision-Language Foundation Models?

Doanh C. Bui(✉), Hoai Luan Pham, Vu Trung Duong Le, Tuan Hai Vu, Van Duy Tran, and Yasuhiko Nakashima

Nara Institute of Science and Technology, Ikoma, Japan
bui.cao_doanh.bd2@naist.ac.jp

Abstract. Lifelong learning for whole-slide images (WSIs) poses the challenge of training a unified model to perform multiple WSI-related tasks, such as cancer subtyping and tumor classification, in a distributed, continual fashion. This is a practical and applicable problem in clinics and hospitals, as WSIs are large, require storage, processing, and transfer time. Training new models whenever new tasks are defined is time-consuming. Recent work has applied regularization- and rehearsal-based methods to this setting. However, the rise of vision-language foundation models that align diagnostic text with pathology images raises the question: *are these models alone sufficient for lifelong WSI learning using zero-shot classification, or is further investigation into continual-learning strategies needed to improve performance?* The empirical study demonstrates that a well-pretrained pathology vision-language foundation model, when used with a simple zero-shot approach, can achieve competitive performance compared to training-based rehearsal and regularization-based continual learning methods. To our knowledge, this is the first study to compare conventional continual-learning approaches with vision-language zero-shot classification for WSIs. Our source code and experimental results will be available at https://github.com/caodoanh2001/ZeroSlide.

Keywords: lifelong learning · whole slide image analysis · pathology vision-language foundation model

1 Introduction

Whole-slide images (WSIs) are gigapixel in size and provide visualization of tissue at the cellular level, playing a key role in cancer diagnosis and prognosis [1]. Computational tools have been developed to support diagnostic tasks such as cancer subtyping [2], tumor classification [3,4], cancer grading [5,6], and survival

N. Akash et al. (Eds.): EMERGE 2025 Workshops, LNCS 16534, pp. 24–33, 2026.
https://doi.org/10.1007/978-3-032-24182-5_3

analysis [7,8]. However, the rapid growth in WSI volume has led to an increasing number of related tasks. Moreover, because WSIs are so large, they require substantial storage, processing, and transfer time. Therefore, it is necessary to investigate how to extend a unified computational model to new WSI-related tasks without retraining or building a new model to save time and effort.

Prior studies on lifelong learning primarily fall into two categories: regularization- and rehearsal-based methods [9–14]. Regularization-based methods constrain the parameters learned on the current task to remain close to those of previous tasks. Notable examples include LwF [9] and EWC [10]. Rehearsal-based methods maintain a fixed-size buffer of representative samples from past tasks for replay during new-task training; examples include ER-ACE [12], AGEM [13], and DER++ [14]. In WSI analysis, ConSlide [15] introduced BuRo, a buffer strategy that partitions slides into regions and randomly recombines them to diversify the buffer without increasing its capacity. Subsequently, [16] proposed a distance consistency loss that minimizes the discrepancy between pairwise distances of current replay sample representations and those stored in a memory bank, thereby stabilizing the replay queue.

Concurrently, MI-Zero [17] introduced a similarity computation between vision features and class prompts for zero-shot classification of WSI tasks following self-supervised contrastive learning, yielding promising results. Foundation pathology vision-language models, such as CONCH [18] and TITAN [19], have been developed using self-supervised methods to align slide embeddings with diagnostic text. These models further strengthen zero-shot classification by matching pathology visual features with text prompts (Fig. 1).

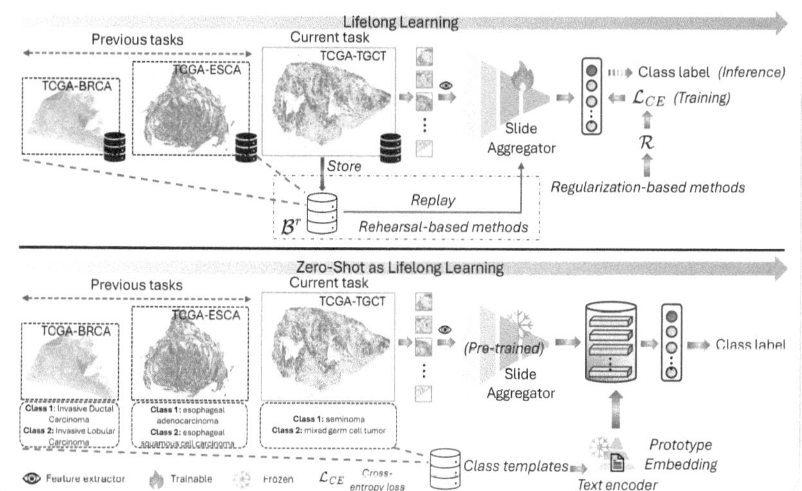

Fig. 1. Regularization-based and rehearsal-based methods require retraining when adding tasks, while zero-shot classification with a pathology vision-language model only needs new class templates, making it training-free. This study compares the performance of lifelong learning with training-free zero-shot classification to training-based continual learning methods.

Given these developments, we pose the following research question: *Is zero-shot classification sufficient for lifelong learning on WSIs when leveraging an advanced pathology vision-language foundation model, or are additional continual learning techniques required?* If zero-shot classification is treated as a lifelong learning method, adding a new task requires only defining a new class text prompt and using a pathology-specific vision-language foundation model to extract text embeddings as a classifier, rather than performing time-consuming continual learning. In this study, we frame zero-shot classification as a lifelong learning approach and compare it head-to-head with training-based continual learning methods on WSI analysis tasks to determine whether zero-shot classification suffices or if continual learning methods still offer superior performance. Our experiments, designed to answer this question, reveal that zero-shot classification is *highly competitive* with continual-learning-based models.

2 Experimental Designs

2.1 Problem Definition

We define the lifelong learning problem for WSI analysis as follows. Let $\mathcal{D} = \{D_i\}_{i=1}^{N}$ be a sequence of N tasks or datasets. Each D_i is partitioned into $D_i = D_i^{\text{train}} \cup D_i^{\text{test}}$, where D_i^{train} is used for training and D_i^{test} for evaluation. After training on the t-th task using D_t^{train}, the algorithm $\mathcal{F}$ must maintain its performance on $\{D_i^{\text{test}}\}_{i<t}$, minimizing forgetting as much as possible. Our objective is to evaluate: (1) whether **zero-shot classification** alone suffices to develop $\mathcal{F}$, or: (2) whether **continual learning approaches**, where $\mathcal{F}$ is trained with techniques designed to mitigate forgetting, are required. Following the evaluation settings of continual learning studies [13–15], there are two scenarios: **class-incremental (CLASS-IL)** and **task-incremental (TASK-IL)**. CLASS-IL requires the model to correctly predict the true class label across all accumulated classes as the number of tasks grows, whereas TASK-IL considers only the logits for the current task's classes. Hence, CLASS-IL is more challenging.

2.2 WSI Tiling and Feature Extraction

Given a WSI, we tile it into K patches using the segmentation and patching strategy of CLAM [3]. We then use the vision-language foundation model TITAN's vision encoder [19] to extract features for each patch. This yields a sequence of patch features $\mathbf{x} = \{x_i\}_{i=1}^{K}$, where $x_i \in \mathbb{R}^{C_{\text{vis}}}$ is a C_{vis}-dimensional feature vector. The sequence $\mathbf{x}$ then undergoes a slide aggregation function $f_{\mathcal{A}}$ to obtain a single slide embedding for classification. To incorporate continual learning, $f_{\mathcal{A}}$ is learnable, and we use HIT [15], which leverages the pyramid structure of a WSI. For zero-shot classification, $f_{\mathcal{A}}$ is pretrained and requires no further training when adapting to new tasks.

2.3 Lifelong Learning for WSIs Using Continual Learning-Based Models

For the regularization-based model, we include Elastic Weight Consolidation (EwC) [10], which leverages parameters from the $(t-1)$-th task's model θ_{t-1} to regularize training of the current model θ_t. EwC [10] approximates the posterior importance of each parameter by a Gaussian centered at θ_{t-1} with precision given by the diagonal of the Fisher information matrix F, then adds a quadratic penalty to prevent important parameters from drifting. These techniques mitigate forgetting by constraining updates to directions deemed critical for previous tasks.

For rehearsal-based models, we select Dark Experience Replay (DER++), a widely used rehearsal-based method, and ConSlide [15], specifically designed for continual learning on WSIs. DER++ performs knowledge distillation by aligning the prediction logits of the current model $f_t^{(i)}$ at iteration i with those of a past model $f_t^{(k)}$ for $k < i$, thereby reducing forgetting. ConSlide proposes a hierarchical transformer to leverage the pyramid structure of WSIs and introduces the BuRo strategy, which breaks a WSI into regions, stores them in a buffer, and then randomly merges them to form new WSIs for replay. For continual learning-based methods, the slide aggregator $f_{\mathcal{A}}$ is trainable and includes a classification head to generate logits.

2.4 Lifelong Learning as WSI Zero-Shot Classification

To formulate lifelong learning as zero-shot classification, we first create a set of class templates for each test dataset D_i^{test}. Following the zero-shot setup of [17], we define $T = 22$ base templates (e.g., "`a histopathological image showing [CLASS].`") and generate ≈ 4 phrasing variants per class. For a dataset with m classes, this yields about $4m$ sentences per class and a total of $\approx 88m$ prompts. We denote the jth class's prompts collectively as c_j, and set $C_i = \{c_j\}_{j=1}^m$. Each prompt in C_i is fed into a text encoder of TITAN vision-language foundation model $f_{\text{text}}^{\text{TITAN}}$, and we average the resulting embeddings across variants to obtain one prototype embedding per class.

ZeroSlide: Adapt To Lifelong Learning. Algorithm 1 details how these embeddings are used for zero-shot classification in the lifelong learning setting. First, a global set of prototypes $\mathcal{T}$ is defined. For each new i-th task, we define its class templates C_i and obtain their embeddings via $f_{\text{text}}^{\text{TITAN}}$. Given test patch features $\mathbf{x}_j \in D_i^{\text{test}}$, we aggregate them into a slide embedding s_i and compute its similarity to each prototype. The prototype with the highest similarity to s_i determines the predicted cancer subtype. In the CLASS-IL scenario, s_i is compared against all prototypes in $\mathcal{T}$; in the TASK-IL scenario, it is compared only to the prototypes of the current task.

We refer to the strategy to adapt zero-shot classification as lifelong learning as **ZeroSlide**.

Algorithm 1. ZeroSlide: Lifelong Learning as WSI Zero-Shot Classification

Input: Sequence of test datasets $\mathcal{D}^{\text{test}} = \{D_i^{\text{test}}\}^{|\mathcal{D}|}$, class templates $\mathcal{C} = \{C_i\}_{i=1}^{|\mathcal{D}|}$
Output: Predicted class label
Initialize: Set of prototype embeddings $\mathcal{T} = \varnothing$
Supporting Operations: TITAN text encoder: $f_{\text{text}}^{\text{TITAN}}$, pre-trained slide encoder: $f_{\mathcal{A}}$

for D_i^{test} **in** $\mathcal{D}^{\text{test}}$ **do**
  $T_i \leftarrow \{f_{\text{text}}^{\text{TITAN}}(c_k) \mid c_k \in C_i\}_{k=1}^{|C_i|}$
    ▷ Extract text embeddings for the i-th task, where $T_i \in \mathbb{R}^{|C_i| \times \text{dim}}$
  $\mathcal{T} \leftarrow \mathcal{T} \cup T_i$ ▷ Add to the text-based classifier, where $\mathcal{T} \in \mathbb{R}^{\sum_{k \le t} |C_k| \times \text{dim}}$
  for $\mathbf{x}_j$ **in** D_i^{test} **do**
    $s_j \leftarrow f_{\mathcal{A}}(\mathbf{x}_j)$ ▷ Aggregate the set of patch features, where $s_j \in \mathbb{R}^{1 \times \text{dim}}$
    $\hat{p}_j^{CI} \leftarrow s_j \odot \mathcal{T}^\top$ ▷ Compute CLASS-IL similarity, where $\hat{p}_j^{CI} \in \mathbb{R}^{1 \times \sum_{k \le t} |C_k|}$
    $\hat{p}_j^{TI} \leftarrow s_j \odot T_i^\top$ ▷ Compute TASK-IL similarity, where $\hat{p}_j^{TI} \in \mathbb{R}^{1 \times |C_i|}$
    $\hat{y}_j^{CI} \leftarrow \arg\max \hat{p}_j^{CI}$ ▷ Get CLASS-IL prediction
    $\hat{y}_j^{TI} \leftarrow \arg\max \hat{p}_j^{TI}$ ▷ Get TASK-IL prediction

3 Experiments

3.1 Datasets

We establish a sequence of six TCGA datasets: TCGA-BRCA (breast), TCGA-RCC (kidney), TCGA-NSCLC (lung), TCGA-ESCA (esophagus), TCGA-TGCT (testis), and TCGA-CESC (cervix uteri). Each dataset addresses a cancer subtyping task. The dataset details are shown in Fig. 2. Each dataset is split into 10 folds, each comprising a train–validation–test split. All experiments are run on 10 folds to ensure stability. For continual learning–based models, training is performed on D_i^{train}; checkpoints are saved based on performance on the validation set D_i^{val}, and results are reported on D_i^{test}. For ZeroSlide, only D_i^{test} is used for evaluation using Algorithm 1 without training.

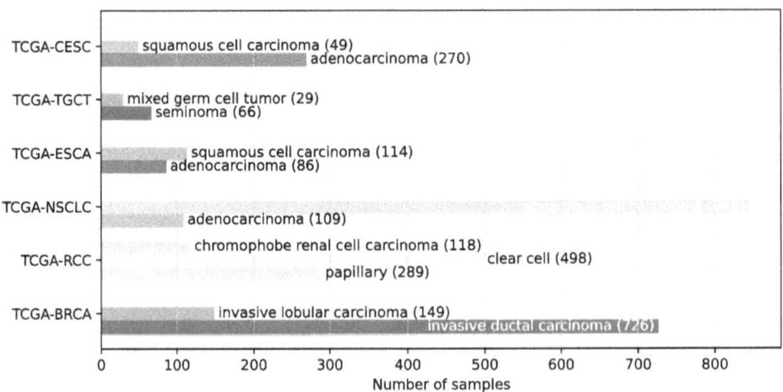

Fig. 2. Distribution of six TCGA datasets.

3.2 Metrics

There are five metrics: Accuracy (ACC), Masked Accuracy (MASKED ACC), Mean Accuracy (mACC), Backward Transfer (BWT), and Forgetting. ACC measures performance under the CLASS-IL scenario using prediction logits $\hat{p}_j^{CI}$ computed with all accumulated prototypes. MASKED ACC measures performance under the Task-IL scenario using prediction logits $\hat{p}_j^{TI}$ computed with prototypes of the current task only. The mACC is the running average of mean task accuracies: after each new task i, compute the mean accuracy over the i tasks seen so far and then average these means across the sequence. BWT quantifies how learning new tasks affects past tasks, indicating positive or negative transfer. Forgetting measures knowledge loss by comparing the highest accuracy achieved on task i with its final accuracy after training on all $|\mathcal{D}|$ datasets/tasks.

3.3 Implemental Details

For all models, we train 10 epochs per task sequentially on six TCGA datasets using the same random seed to ensure stable comparisons. For the backbone $f_{\mathcal{A}}$ used to extract slide embeddings in all continual learning methods, we employ HIT [15], which is designed to aggregate features from the patch to region level. Regions are tiled at 10× magnification into 1024×1024 pixel areas and then each region is cropped into 4 × 4 patches of 256 × 256 pixels. Both patch and region features are obtained using $f_{\text{vis}}^{\text{TITAN}}$, with $C_{\text{vis}} = 768$. For embedding dimension in HIT, we use $dim = 384$.

3.4 Experimental Results

Main Results. The results, reported in Table 1, reveal an interesting finding: despite being training-free, *ZeroSlide achieves competitive performance with rehearsal-based continual learning methods DER++ and ConSlide, and significantly outperforms the regularization-based method EWC.* For rehearsal-based methods, with a buffer size of $|\mathcal{B}_r| = 30$, ConSlide attains the highest ACC in the CLASS-IL scenario (65.673 %) and the second-best Masked ACC in the TASK-IL scenario (90.255 %), as well as mACC (82.602 %). These margins over ZeroSlide are small (+1.544 % ACC, +0.497 % Masked ACC, and +0.009 % mACC). Furthermore, ZeroSlide outperforms DER++ (with $|\mathcal{B}_r| = 10$ or 30) in ACC by +5.131 % and +7.510 %, respectively, although DER++ still leads in TASK-IL. We also observe that *ZeroSlide is more stable with respect to the BWT and Forgetting metrics.* Regarding Forgetting, ZeroSlide achieves the best score (0.909), while securing the second-best BWT (âĂŞ0.909). These results suggest that advanced training-based WSI-specific continual learning models still outperform ZeroSlide in CLASS-IL accuracy. However, adapting zero-shot classification to lifelong learning is both promising and feasible, as ZeroSlide's performance remains not only highly competitive with training-based continual learning methods under both CLASS-IL and TASK-IL scenarios but also demonstrates the most stability in BWT and Forgetting metrics.

Table 1. Experimental results on a sequence of six TCGA datasets. Red highlights the best performance, while blue highlights the second-best.

Method	Buffer size $\|\mathcal{B}_r\|$	ACC	MASKED ACC	mACC	BWT ↑	Forgetting ↓
Regularization-based Methods (Training-based)						
EWC	0	43.522 (±6.765)	89.244 (±1.902)	69.834 (±3.566)	-3.617 (±3.101)	4.649 (±2.558)
Rehearsal-based Methods (Training-based)						
DER++	≈ 10	56.619 (±4.027)	89.571 (±1.051)	81.786 (±1.575)	-3.627 (±1.182)	4.266 (±1.089)
ConSlide	≈ 10	64.226 (±4.282)	89.318 (±2.349)	81.992 (±1.055)	0.196 (±1.745)	4.849 (±2.527)
DER++	≈ 30	58.998 (±1.219)	90.604 (±1.472)	83.580 (±1.532)	-2.368 (±1.889)	3.199 (±1.640)
ConSlide	≈ 30	65.673 (±1.780)	90.255 (±1.334)	82.602 (±1.201)	-2.930 (±1.506)	4.032 (±1.248)
Lifelong Learning as Zero-Shot Classification (Training-free)						
ZeroSlide	0	64.129 (±1.591)	89.758 (±0.984)	82.593 (±0.017)	-0.909 (±0.406)	0.909 (±0.406)

Confidence Score Study. We examine the prediction results of all models to investigate the stability of predictions across tasks after training the final task, as shown in Fig. 3. We analyze the prediction scores corresponding to the ground-truth labels to assess the model's confidence in the true labels. For ZeroSlide, we consider all scores computed with prototypes in $\mathcal{T}$. For the other three models, we examine the logits across all cancer subtypes in $|\mathcal{D}|$ datasets/tasks after softmax. Our first observation is that ZeroSlide's score is significantly lower than the other continual learning models. This is expected, as ZeroSlide is training-free and uses class template prototypes while distance between the slide embedding and the prototype is not perfectly close. For the training-based models, the score with the target label is high. However, EWC shows significant degradation in confidence for TCGA-BRCA (median ≈ 0.1) and TCGA-RCC (median ≈ 0.3) as tasks increase, while DER++ and ConSlide maintain high performance on these datasets (median ≥ 0.75). All models struggle with TCGA-ESCA test samples, with extremely low confidence scores. EWC and DER++ even achieve a median confidence score of 0 on TCGA-ESCA, while ZeroSlide has a median of ≈ 0.09. EWC and DER++ also show low confidence for TGCT. Overall, ConSlide demonstrates the best stability in confidence as tasks increase. While ZeroSlide's scores with target prototypes are modest, they are still sufficiently sensitive to correctly classify cancer subtypes, making its performance highly competitive with ConSlide and other continual learning models.

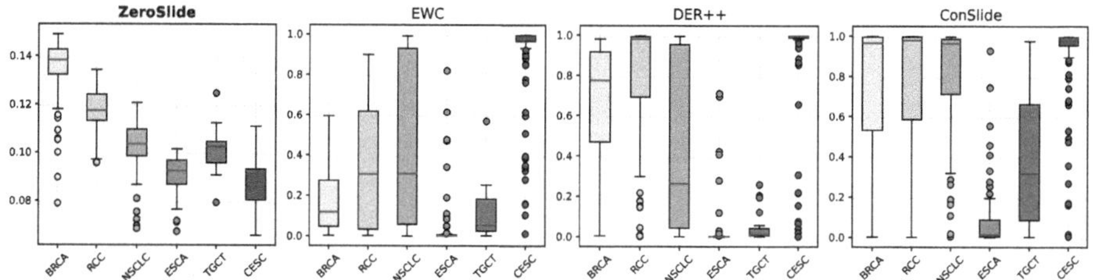

Fig. 3. Confidence scores for target cancer subtype labels after training/inference on the final tasks of ZeroSlide and all continual-learning-based models.

4 Discussion

Based on the experimental designs and results, we conclude that *leveraging advanced pathology vision-language foundation models and performing zero-shot classification is feasible for lifelong WSI analysis* in two key ways: 1) ZeroSlide's performance asymptotically matches or surpasses continual learning methods, and 2) it is fully training-free, requiring no storage for WSIs. Despite these promising results, we highlight the limitations of ZeroSlide and suggest future improvements for lifelong learning.

Risk of Ambiguous Class Prediction. As shown in Fig. 3, ZeroSlide's confidence score for the target label is significantly lower than that of DER++ and ConSlide. This indicates that if class templates are poorly defined or if tasks include out-of-distribution class names, ZeroSlide may not perform effectively in a lifelong learning setting.

Perspectives for Improvement. Although ZeroSlide is effective, training-based continual learning methods still yield strong results. Future work could involve integrating class templates with methods like ConSlide to enhance performance. The CATE approach [20] maximizes informative features using text prompts but requires time and storage for class template embeddings during inference. A promising direction would be to limit class prompt usage to online training, ignoring it during inference. Additionally, current continual learning methods require training over multiple epochs when new tasks are added. An ideal approach would involve leveraging class templates from pathology vision-language foundation models to minimize training epochs.

5 Conclusion

This study examines zero-shot classification using a pathology vision-language foundation model (ZeroSlide) and compares it with training-based continual learning methods for lifelong WSI analysis. Experimental results across six TCGA datasets suggest that ZeroSlide performs similarly to continual learning models, while being training-free and incurring no storage or online buffer costs.

However, some limitations are noted, and future studies are recommended to improve lifelong learning for WSIs. We believe this study bridges the knowledge gap in zero-shot classification within the pathology vision-language model era and encourages developments to make lifelong learning for WSI analysis more applicable and practical in clinical settings.

Acknowledgments. This work was supported in part by the Japan Science and Technology Agency (JST)-Advanced Technologies for CArbon-Neutral (ALCA-Next)-Next Program, Japan, under Grant JPMJAN23F4; in part by the Japan Society for the Promotion of Science (JSPS), Grants-in-Aid for Scientific Research (KAKENHI), Japan, under Grant 22H00515; and in part by the Next Generation Researchers Challenging Research Program under Grant zk25010020.

Disclosure of Interests. The authors declare that they have no conflict of interest.

References

1. Wu, S., Hong, G., Xu, A., et al.: Artificial intelligence-based model for lymph node metastases detection on whole slide images in bladder cancer: a retrospective, multicentre, diagnostic study. Lancet Oncol. **24**(4), 360–370 (2023)
2. Zhang, H., Meng, Y., Zhao, Y., et al.: "DTFD-MIL: double-tier feature distillation multiple instance learning for histopathology whole slide image classification. In: Proceedings of the IEEE/CVF Conference on Computer Vision and Pattern Recognition, pp. 18802–18812 (2022)
3. Lu, M.Y., Williamson, D.F., Chen, T.Y., Chen, R.J., Barbieri, M., Mahmood, F.: Data-efficient and weakly supervised computational pathology on whole-slide images. Nat. Biomed. Eng. **5**(6), 555–570 (2021)
4. Shao, Z., Bian, H., Chen, Y., Wang, Y., Zhang, J., Ji, X., et al.: Transmil: transformer based correlated multiple instance learning for whole slide image classification. Adv. Neural. Inf. Process. Syst. **34**, 2136–2147 (2021)
5. Le Vuong, T.T., Kim, K., Song, B., Kwak, J.T.: Joint categorical and ordinal learning for cancer grading in pathology images. Med. Image Anal. **73**, 102206 (2021)
6. Bui, D.C., Song, B., Kim, K., Kwak, J.T.: Spatially-constrained and unconstrained bi-graph interaction network for multi-organ pathology image classification. IEEE Trans. Med. Imaging (2024)
7. Li, R., Yao, J., Zhu, X., Li, Y., Huang, J.: Graph CNN for survival analysis on whole slide pathological images. In: Frangi, A.F., Schnabel, J.A., Davatzikos, C., Alberola-López, C., Fichtinger, G. (eds.) MICCAI 2018. LNCS, vol. 11071, pp. 174–182. Springer, Cham (2018). https://doi.org/10.1007/978-3-030-00934-2_20
8. Liu, P., Ji, L., Ye, F., Fu, B.: Advmil: adversarial multiple instance learning for the survival analysis on whole-slide images. Med. Image Anal. **91**, 103020 (2024)
9. Li, Z., Hoiem, D.: Learning without forgetting. IEEE Trans. Pattern Anal. Mach. Intell. **40**(12), 2935–2947 (2017)
10. Kirkpatrick, J., Pascanu, R., Rabinowitz, N., et al.: Overcoming catastrophic forgetting in neural networks. Proc. Natl. Acad. Sci. **114**(13), 3521–3526 (2017)
11. Prabhu, A., Torr, P.H.S., Dokania, P.K.: GDumb: a simple approach that questions our progress in continual learning. In: Vedaldi, A., Bischof, H., Brox, T., Frahm, J.-M. (eds.) ECCV 2020. LNCS, vol. 12347, pp. 524–540. Springer, Cham (2020). https://doi.org/10.1007/978-3-030-58536-5_31

12. Caccia, L., Aljundi, R., Asadi, N., Tuytelaars, T., Pineau, J., Belilovsky, E.: New insights on reducing abrupt representation change in online continual learning. arXiv preprint arXiv:2104.05025 (2021)
13. Chaudhry, A., Ranzato, M., Rohrbach, M., Elhoseiny, M.: Efficient lifelong learning with a-gem. arXiv preprint arXiv:1812.00420 (2018)
14. Buzzega, P., Boschini, M., Porrello, A., Abati, D., Calderara, S.: Dark experience for general continual learning: a strong, simple baseline. Adv. Neural. Inf. Process. Syst. **33**, 15920–15930 (2020)
15. Huang, Y., Zhao, W., Wang, S., Fu, Y., Jiang, Y., Yu, L.: Conslide: asynchronous hierarchical interaction transformer with breakup-reorganize rehearsal for continual whole slide image analysis. In: Proceedings of the IEEE/CVF International Conference on Computer Vision, pp. 21349–21360 (2023)
16. Zhu, X., Jiang, Z., Wu, K., Shi, J., Zheng, Y.: Lifelong histopathology whole slide image retrieval via distance consistency rehearsal. In: International Conference on Medical Image Computing and Computer-Assisted Intervention, pp. 274–284. Springer, Cham (2024). https://doi.org/10.1007/978-3-031-72083-3_26
17. Lu, M.Y., Chen, B., Zhang, A., et al.: Visual language pretrained multiple instance zero-shot transfer for histopathology images. In: Proceedings of the IEEE/CVF Conference on Computer Vision and Pattern Recognition, pp. 19764–19775 (2023)
18. Lu, M.Y., Chen, B., Williamson, D.F., et al.: A visual-language foundation model for computational pathology. Nat. Med. **30**(3), 863–874 (2024)
19. Ding, T., Wagner, S.J., Song, A.H., et al.: Multimodal whole slide foundation model for pathology. arXiv preprint arXiv:2411.19666 (2024)
20. Huang, Y., Zhao, W., Chen, Y., Fu, Y., Yu, L.: Free lunch in pathology foundation model: Task-specific model adaptation with concept-guided feature enhancement. Adv. Neural. Inf. Process. Syst. **37**, 79963–79995 (2024)

Oral Presentations 2: Representation Learning for Detection and Diagnosis

GroundingDINO for Open-Set Lesion Detection in Medical Imaging

Samuel J. Roughley[1(✉)], Johanna P. Müller[2], Shangqi Gao[3,4], Zeyu Gao[3,4], Marta Ligero[5], Rudolfs Blums[6], Mireia Crispin-Ortuzar[3,4], Julia Schnabel[6,7,8,9], Bernhard Kainz[2,10], Cosmin I. Bercea[6,7], and Ines Prata Machado[3,4]

[1] Department of Physics, University of Cambridge, Cambridge, UK
sjr220@cantab.ac.uk
[2] Friedrich-Alexander University Erlangen-Nürnberg, Erlangen, Germany
[3] Department of Oncology, University of Cambridge, Cambridge, UK
[4] Early Cancer Institute, University of Cambridge, Cambridge, UK
[5] Else Kroener Fresenius Center for Digital Health, Technical University Dresden, Dresden, Germany
[6] Technical University of Munich, Munich, Germany
[7] Helmholtz AI and Helmholtz Center Munich, Munich, Germany
[8] Munich Center for Machine Learning, Munich, Germany
[9] King's College London, London, UK
[10] Imperial College London, London, UK

Abstract. Open-world anomaly detection is a task in which machine learning is well-positioned to advance cancer diagnosis, potentially leading to significantly improved survival rates. For a model to be used in clinical settings, it must demonstrate high performance, robustness, and generalisability. A common approach to achieving high generalisability is to incorporate information from broader representations within the model. In this work, we investigate the application of GroundingDINO to medical anomaly detection and localisation, evaluating both its overall performance and the influence of text prompts. We find that GroundingDINO outperforms the YOLOv11n model even with minimal use of contextual information. When exploring methods to introduce more contextual information, we observe that specifying the organ within the prompt improves closed-set performance on rarer lesion classes. However, adding visual descriptions of lesions during training leads to a significant performance drop on those subsets, indicating that the model memorises prompt-image pairs rather than learning meaningful semantic relationships. Our work highlights a critical limitation of GroundingDINO in medical imaging and proposes targeted modifications to the model architecture or training strategies as promising directions for utilising richer semantic prompts to improve anomaly detection.

Keywords: Anomaly Detection · GroundingDINO · Prompt Engineering · Medical Imaging · Lesion Detection · Cancer Research

N. Akash et al. (Eds.): EMERGE 2025 Workshops, LNCS 16534, pp. 37–46, 2026.
https://doi.org/10.1007/978-3-032-24182-5_4

1 Introduction

Early detection is critical to improving survival outcomes for cancer, which accounts for nearly 1 in 6 deaths globally [14,16]. To aid in diagnosis, medical imaging technologies such as Computed Tomography (CT) and Magnetic Resonance Imaging (MRI) provide detailed 3D anatomical views. However, automated identification of open-world anomalies in these scans has not kept pace with advancements in imaging technologies, as interpreting the resulting images remains highly challenging [17]. For example, studies have found that approximately one-third of diagnoses are often missed across various diagnostic pathways [3,8]. Therefore, research into computer-aided cancer detection is invaluable not only for improving cancer survival rates but also for alleviating the growing burden on healthcare systems. As such, significant effort has been dedicated to developing machine learning models for medical anomaly detection (AD). The appearance of cancer varies widely across types, subtypes, and individual patients, making robust open-set performance challenging [7,20]. However, for a model to be clinically viable, it must be capable of detecting both common and rare, or previously unseen, pathologies. A common strategy for improving generalisability is to incorporate contextual information into the model. For example, the GroundingDINO model achieves state-of-the-art open-set performance in the natural imaging domain by introducing language prompts into a closed-set detector [11]. Despite such successes, however, these methods remain relatively underexplored in the medical domain. **Contributions.** We present the first investigation of GroundingDINO for medical anomaly detection, focusing on lesion detection in CT scans of the chest-abdomen-pelvis region, and compare its performance with the state-of-the-art YOLOv11n model. Through a series of experiments using varied text prompts, we examine the impact of prompt design on both closed-set and open-set performance, exploring how semantic information can enhance medical AD. Our ultimate goal is to lay the groundwork for future integration of text and image modalities to achieve state-of-the-art performance with real clinical applicability.

2 Methodology

Background. GroundingDINO is a transformer-based vision-language model originally trained for object detection on natural images. Its primary goal is to generalise to unseen object classes by integrating semantic information via language into the closed-set detector DINO [21], thereby enabling open-set capabilities. The model's architecture includes three cross-modality fusion points, which the authors argue provide stronger language guidance during detection compared to models with fewer fusion locations [11]. Open-set detection is particularly relevant in medical imaging tasks such as cancer screening, where rare and previously unseen lesions may be encountered. Recent work has highlighted the importance of integrating semantic priors to improve detection generalisation in these settings [2]. Recent advances in Large Language Models (LLMs),

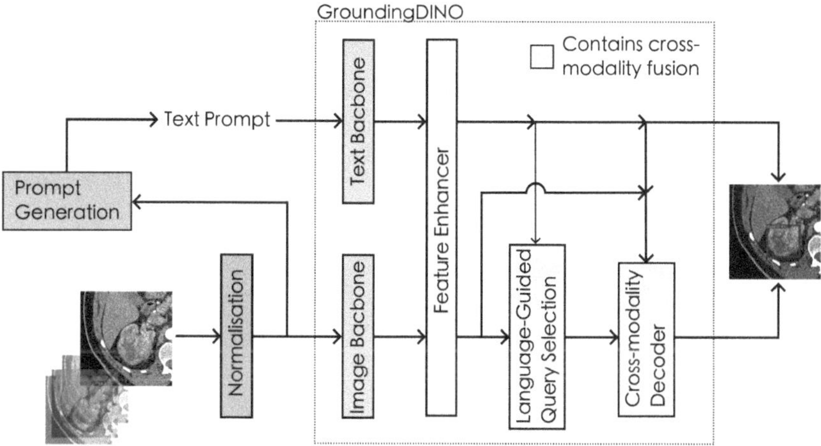

Fig. 1. Detection pipeline used during experiments, highlighting the inclusion of the GroundingDINO architecture. A single slice is normalised and a text prompt generated, before being passed to GroundingDINO to perform the detection. The locations of cross-modality fusion are highlighted: cross-attention blocks within the feature enhancer and decoder, and language guidance of query selection. Multiple methods for prompt generation were explored, so it is shown generally.

such as Gemini [18], BiomedGPT [13], and ChatGPT-4 [1], have demonstrated strong capabilities in generating clinically rich, context-aware descriptions. These models provide a powerful means of constructing descriptive prompts to guide open-set detection models in medical applications [12]. Despite its comparatively modest size and training data, GroundingDINO achieves state-of-the-art performance on open-set detection benchmarks, outperforming larger models such as GLIP [9] in the COCO zero-shot setting [10]. Its utility in medical contexts has already been demonstrated in the BiomedParse study [22], where it was used to propose bounding boxes without additional training.

Model Architecture. The pipeline used in our experiments is illustrated in Fig. 1. Since GroundingDINO is limited to 2D detection, a single slice must first be selected from the scan. The slice is then normalised to improve consistency across samples. Before being passed to GroundingDINO, a text prompt must also be generated. As the method of prompt generation varies across our experiments, a general representation is shown in Fig. 1. When relevant, the images are used post-normalisation to generate the prompts. The prompt and normalised image are then passed to the GroundingDINO architecture, where the text and image backbones extract features from the inputs. The feature enhancer then updates the features, making use of text-to-image and image-to-text cross-attention. The updated text features then guide the selection of queries to be used in the decoder, where text and image cross-attention are used to generate the model outputs. For additional details, we refer the reader to the original work by Liu et al. [11]

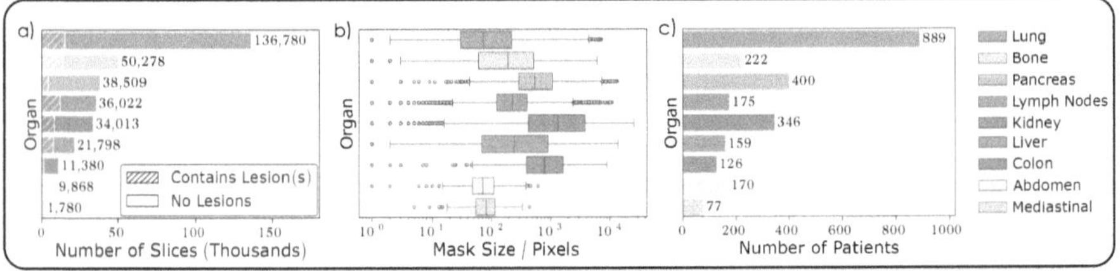

Fig. 2. Breakdown of the ULS23 Dataset. a) Number of slices from scans containing (no) lesions in each organ. b) Distribution of mask sizes by organ, with samples outside 1.5 times the IQR from the nearest quartile shown as outliers. c) Number of patients with scans of lesions in each organ.

3 Evaluation

Datasets. For training and evaluation, we used the Universal Lesion Segmentation Challenge 2023 (ULS23) dataset [5], comprising chest-abdomen-pelvic CT scans with segmentation mask annotations. The dataset contains 6,382 lesions from 2,627 patients across various organs (Fig. 2). Each scan is cropped to a volume of interest (VOI) of $256 \times 256 \times 128$ voxels, centred on a single annotated lesion. Although lesion centring introduces bias, this controlled setup establishes baseline performance. Extending to whole-volume detection is required for clinical use and can be addressed in future translation work.

Pre-processing. Annotations of multiple lesions from the same scan were combined into a single annotation without merging adjacent lesions, enabling detection use. Segmentation masks were converted to bounding boxes for GroundingDINO. Scans were normalised first. Due to wide variation in Hounsfield units (HU) across lesions, fixed windowing was unsuitable. Following the ULS23 baseline, Z-score normalisation was applied per slice. Visibility–measured as the absolute difference between median lesion and surrounding intensities divided by local standard deviation–improved for all lesion types except those in bone, indicating potential bias. The dataset was split into 80% training (274,617 slices), 10% validation (33,995 slices), and 10% testing (36,230 slices), with organ-specific and patient-level separation to prevent data leakage.

Experiments. Three experiment types were conducted with models trained on prompts of varying detail. The first used a simple prompt, *"lesion"*, for all scans, providing minimal language guidance and serving as a baseline. Equivalent YOLOv11n models [6], which lack language input, were trained for comparison, mainly relevant to this first experiment. The second experiment specified the organ in the prompt (e.g., *"[organ] lesion"*). The third fine-tuned these models using visual descriptions generated by Gemini ('gemini-2.5-pro-preview-03-25' model) [18], focusing on lymph node lesions due to their moderate sample size and lower initial performance. All three experiments were run both with all lesion types and with mediastinal lesions (4,879 training slices) excluded, as they had

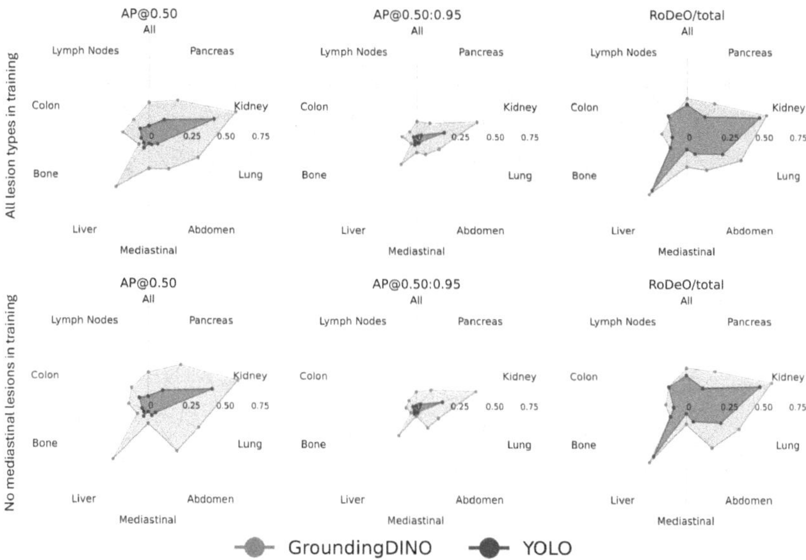

Fig. 3. Radar charts comparing the performance of GroundingDINO and YOLO stratified by organ, with the prompt of *"lesion"* given to GroundingDINO. Average Precision and RoDeO/total metrics are shown for GroundingDINO (green) and YOLO (blue) models that saw all lesion types (top) and all except mediastinal lesions (bottom) from the ULS23 dataset during training.

the fewest samples, minimising training set reduction. Testing on excluded mediastinal lesions evaluates open-set performance. Since data consists of cropped CT scans, each shows only a small anatomical region.

Training Strategy. To train GroundingDINO, the Open-GroundingDINO training code was used with default model hyperparameters and data augmentations [23]. The released GroundingDINO model with the Swin-T image backbone was used as the initialization, and bert-base-uncased [4] from Hugging Face [19] served as the text backbone. For YOLO training, the default implementation from the Ultralytics Python package was used. All models were trained for 25 epochs on NVIDIA A40 and L40S GPUs. To evaluate model performance, we used the Average Precision (AP) and RoDeO [15] metrics. For RoDeO, a bounding box threshold of 0.2 was selected based on sweeps over the validation set.

4 Results

4.1 Minimal Language Guidance

The results for the GroundingDINO models using the prompt *"lesion"* for all scans, along with the corresponding YOLO models, are shown in Fig. 3. GroundingDINO performs as well as or better than YOLO across all organs. GroundingDINO's superior performance using only simple prompts indicates

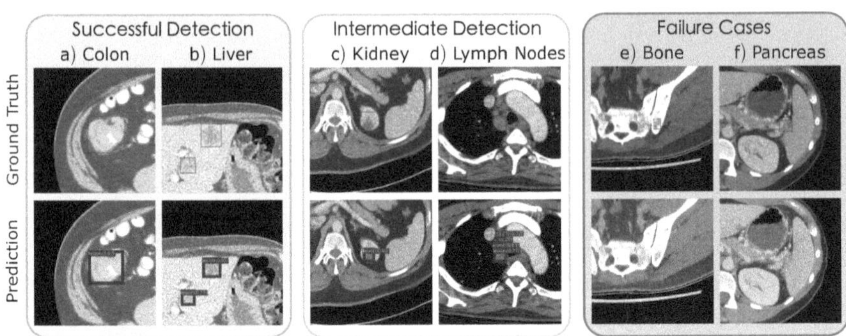

Fig. 4. Inference examples from the GroundingDINO model trained on lesions across all organs in the ULS23 dataset, using *"lesion"* as the text prompt. Ground truth annotations (top, red boxes) and model predictions (bottom, blue boxes) are shown for six organ sites.

that semantic alignment, not present in YOLO, offers tangible benefits independent of prompt complexity, highlighting the model's potential suitability for medical anomaly detection and supporting its use in research such as ours. Inference examples from the GroundingDINO model trained on all lesion types are shown in Fig. 4, illustrating both successful detections and failure cases. Figure 4c highlights ambiguities in lesion definition, bounding an internal substructure within the ground truth. Figure 4d contains false positives, typically observed near anatomical features resembling lesion morphology (e.g., vessels or bones). The issue of false positives is noted in the original GroundingDINO paper [11]. The persistence of these issues with minimal prompts points to the need for more precise annotations and improved semantic grounding. As expected, after removing mediastinal lesions from training, performance on mediastinal lesions drops significantly. However, while YOLO's performance falls to near zero (e.g., RoDeO/total = 0.013), GroundingDINO maintains better performance. This better preservation of accuracy, even before introducing additional language guidance, suggests stronger inherent generalisability, making results especially relevant in discussions of clinical deployment. Nevertheless, the sizeable performance drop underscores that open-set detection remains a significant challenge. Consequently, with multimodal models like GroundingDINO, it is natural to consider whether language guidance can mitigate this decline.

4.2 Enhanced Language Guidance

The results for the different GroundingDINO models using the three different prompt types are shown in Fig. 5.

Organ-Specific Prompts. Organ-specific prompts show no definitive overall effect on performance. A slight improvement is seen when all organs are included in training, but its small magnitude and disappearance when mediastinal lesions

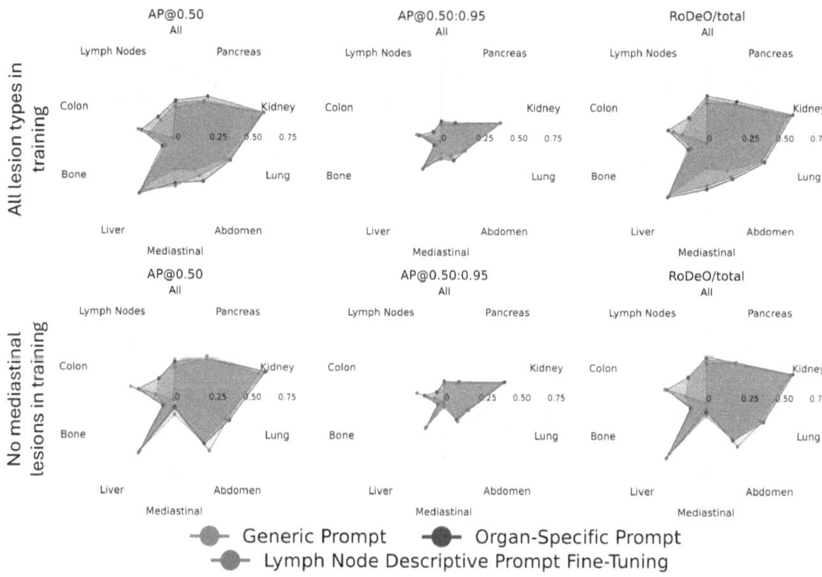

Fig. 5. Radar charts comparing the performance of GroundingDINO models stratified by organ, with the models differing by the choice of text prompt used. Average Precision and RoDeO/total metrics are shown for GroundingDINO models that saw all lesion types (top) and all except mediastinal lesions (bottom) from the ULS23 dataset during training. Prompts of *"lesion"* (green), *"[organ] lesion"* (blue) and the addition of visual descriptions (red) were all tested.

are excluded make its significance unclear. Notably, performance improves for colon (54% RoDeO/total), mediastinal (87%), and abdominal (30%) lesions when all lesion types are included. These gains likely result from limited training data for these lesion types (Fig. 2a), making them more susceptible to being overshadowed. Organ-specific prompts reduce interclass competition, helping the model learn relevant visual features. A similar improvement is observed for colon lesions when mediastinal lesions are excluded. However, no gains are seen for mediastinal or abdominal lesions. For mediastinal lesions, this is expected, as the model had no exposure to them. For abdominal lesions, the absence of improvement suggests their performance was suppressed specifically by the presence of mediastinal lesions, despite the latter being the smallest class.

Descriptive Prompts. After fine-tuning models using visual descriptions for lymph node lesions during training, performance on lymph node lesions dropped to zero. In the test set, none of the model's predictions for lymph node lesions exceeded a confidence score of 0.05, explaining why RoDeO/total = 0. To better understand this behaviour, the model outputs were analysed in more detail. During inference, GroundingDINO generates 900 (box, caption) pairs. For each pair, an activation score is computed for every token in the text input, and tokens with scores above a threshold form the caption. Examples of the mean

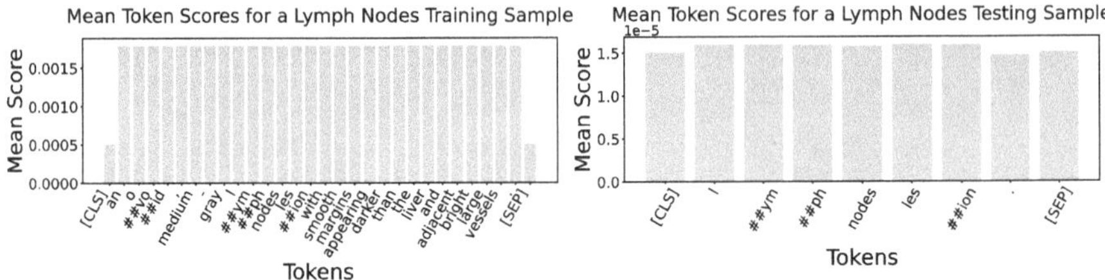

Fig. 6. Token-level activation maps from GroundingDINO for a lymph node lesion sample from the training and testing sets, showing uniformly distributed attention across tokens.

activation scores across the 900 predictions for a training and testing sample are shown in Fig. 6.

Activation is highly uniform across tokens. Excluding start and end markers, the maximum activation difference per prediction is just 0.0001 in training and 0.00004 in testing. GroundingDINO is meant to align text and image features so semantics guide detection, but the uniformity suggests overfitting: the model aligns the entire prompt with image features rather than understanding it. As a result, it fails to link the test prompt "lymph node lesion" to relevant training visuals, leading to inaccurate predictions, especially when training and test prompts differ, which earlier experiments did not reveal. The drop in lymph node performance to zero, despite previous success with descriptive prompts, suggests the initial learning rate was too high. A lower rate might have preserved some understanding but would not fix the uniform activation, which stems from how GroundingDINO learns. Addressing this may require changes to the loss function, text encoder, or prompt engineering.

5 Conclusions

GroundingDINO was found to outperform the YOLOv11n model when prompted with the term *"lesion"*, highlighting its suitability for research into medical anomaly detection. Incorporating organ-specific information into text prompts significantly improves closed-set performance on rare lesion classes, emphasising the importance of semantic conditioning. Although overall and open-set performance remain unchanged, these findings suggest clear opportunities for improvement. Using detailed visual lesion descriptions during training revealed overfitting issues that hinder semantic generalization, underscoring the need to refine training methods to better leverage language-based cues.

Acknowledgments. C.I.B. is funded via the EVUK programme ("Next-generation AI for Integrated Diagnostics") of the Free State of Bavaria and partially supported by the Helmholtz Association [Munich School for Data Science]. This work is also supported by the Berdelle-Stiftung [TimeFlow]. The authors acknowledge scientific support and HPC resources from NHR@FAU [b143dc, b180dc], funded by federal and Bavarian authorities, with partial hardware funding from the DFG [440719683]. Additional support was received from the ERC [101083647], the DFG [KA 5801/2-1, INST 90/1351-1], and the state of Bavaria. Further funding was provided by Cancer Research UK [A22905], the CRUK Cambridge Centre [CTRQQR-2021-100012, A25177], The Mark Foundation for Cancer Research [RG95043], GE HealthCare, the CRUK National Cancer Imaging Translational Accelerator [A27066], and the NIHR Cambridge Biomedical Research Centre [NIHR203312, BRC-1215-20014].

Disclosure of Interest. The authors have no competing interests to declare that are relevant to the content of this article.

References

1. Achiam, J., et al.: Gpt-4 technical report. arXiv preprint arXiv:2303.08774 (2023)
2. Aleem, S., et al.: Test-time adaptation with SALIP: a cascade of SAM and clip for zero-shot medical image segmentation. In: Proceedings of the IEEE/CVF Conference on Computer Vision and Pattern Recognition, pp. 5184–5193 (2024)
3. Berlin, L.: Accuracy of diagnostic procedures: has it improved over the past five decades? Am. J. Roentgenol. **188**(5), 1173–1178 (2007). https://doi.org/10.2214/AJR.06.1270, https://www.ajronline.org/doi/full/10.2214/AJR.06.1270. publisher: American Roentgen Ray Society
4. Devlin, J., Chang, M.W., Lee, K., Toutanova, K.: BERT: pre-training of Deep bidirectional transformers for language understanding (2019). https://doi.org/10.48550/arXiv.1810.04805, http://arxiv.org/abs/1810.04805, arXiv:1810.04805 [cs]
5. Grauw, M.J.J.D., et al.: The ULS23 challenge: a baseline model and benchmark dataset for 3D universal lesion segmentation in computed tomography (2024). https://doi.org/10.48550/arXiv.2406.05231, http://arxiv.org/abs/2406.05231, arXiv:2406.05231
6. Jocher, G., Qiu, J.: Ultralytics yolo11 (2024). https://github.com/ultralytics/ultralytics
7. Khader, A., et al.: Importance of tumor subtypes in cancer imaging. Eur. J. Radiol. Open **9** (2022). https://doi.org/10.1016/j.ejro.2022.100433, https://www.ejropen.com/article/S2352-0477(22)00040-5/fulltext
8. Kim, Y.W., Mansfield, L.T.: Fool me twice: delayed diagnoses in radiology with emphasis on perpetuated errors. Am. J. Roentgenol. **202**(3), 465–470 (2014). https://doi.org/10.2214/AJR.13.11493, https://www.ajronline.org/doi/10.2214/AJR.13.11493Roentgen Ray Society
9. Li, L.H., et al.: Grounded language-image pre-training (2022). https://doi.org/10.48550/arXiv.2112.03857, http://arxiv.org/abs/2112.03857, arXiv:2112.03857
10. Lin, T.-Y., et al.: Microsoft COCO: common objects in context. In: Fleet, D., Pajdla, T., Schiele, B., Tuytelaars, T. (eds.) ECCV 2014. LNCS, vol. 8693, pp. 740–755. Springer, Cham (2014). https://doi.org/10.1007/978-3-319-10602-1_48
11. Liu, S., et al.: Grounding DINO: marrying DINO with grounded pre-training for open-set object detection (2024). https://doi.org/10.48550/arXiv.2303.05499, http://arxiv.org/abs/2303.05499, arXiv:2303.05499
12. Liu, X., et al.: Segment any tissue: One-shot reference guided training-free automatic point prompting for medical image segmentation. Med. Image Anal. **102**, 103550 (2025)
13. Luo, Y., et al.: Biomedgpt: an open multimodal large language model for biomedicine. IEEE J. Biomed. Health Inform. (2024)

14. McPhail, S., Johnson, S., Greenberg, D., Peake, M., Rous, B.: Stage at diagnosis and early mortality from cancer in England. Br. J. Cancer **112**(1), S108–S115 (2015). https://doi.org/10.1038/bjc.2015.49, https://www.nature.com/articles/bjc201549
15. Meissen, F., Müller, P., Kaissis, G., Rueckert, D.: Robust detection outcome: a metric for pathology detection in medical images (2023). https://doi.org/10.48550/arXiv.2303.01920, http://arxiv.org/abs/2303.01920, arXiv:2303.01920 [cs]
16. Organisation, W.H.: Cancer (2022). https://www.who.int/news-room/fact-sheets/detail/cancer. Accessed 20 Nov 2024
17. Robinson, P.J.: Radiology's Achilles' heel: error and variation in the interpretation of the Röntgen image. Br. J. Radiol. **70**(839), 1085–1098 (1997). https://doi.org/10.1259/bjr.70.839.9536897
18. Team, G., et al.: Gemini: a family of highly capable multimodal models (2025). https://doi.org/10.48550/arXiv.2312.11805, http://arxiv.org/abs/2312.11805, arXiv:2312.11805 [cs]
19. Wolf, T., et al.: HuggingFace's transformers: state-of-the-art natural language processing (2020). https://doi.org/10.48550/arXiv.1910.03771, http://arxiv.org/abs/1910.03771, arXiv:1910.03771 [cs]
20. Wu, J., et al.: Identifying relations between imaging phenotypes and molecular subtypes of breast cancer: Model discovery and external validation. J. Magn. Reson. Imaging **46**(4), 1017–1027 (2017). https://doi.org/10.1002/jmri.25661, https://onlinelibrary.wiley.com/doi/abs/10.1002/jmri.25661
21. Zhang, H., et al.: DINO: DETR with Improved DeNoising anchor boxes for end-to-end object detection (2022). https://doi.org/10.48550/arXiv.2203.03605, http://arxiv.org/abs/2203.03605, arXiv:2203.03605
22. Zhao, T., et al.: BiomedParse: a biomedical foundation model for image parsing of everything everywhere all at once. Nat. Methods **22**(1), 166–176 (2025). https://doi.org/10.1038/s41592-024-02499-w, http://arxiv.org/abs/2405.12971, arXiv:2405.12971 [cs]
23. Zuwei Long, W.L.: Open grounding dino:the third party implementation of the paper grounding dino (2023). https://github.com/longzw1997/Open-GroundingDino

Structured Spectral Graph Learning for Anomaly Classification in 3D Chest CT Scans

Theo Di Piazza[1,2(✉)], Carole Lazarus[3], Olivier Nempont[3], and Loic Boussel[1,2]

[1] University of Lyon, INSA Lyon, CNRS, INSERM, CREATIS UMR 5220, U1294, Villeurbanne, France
theo.dipiazza@creatis.insa-lyon.fr

[2] Hospices Civils de Lyon, Lyon, France

[3] Philips Clinical Informatics, Innovation Paris, Paris, France

Abstract. With the increasing number of CT scan examinations, there is a need for automated methods such as organ segmentation, anomaly detection and report generation to assist radiologists in managing their increasing workload. Multi-label classification of 3D CT scans remains a critical yet challenging task due to the complex spatial relationships within volumetric data and the variety of observed anomalies. Existing approaches based on 3D convolutional networks have limited abilities to model long-range dependencies while Vision Transformers suffer from high computational costs and often require extensive pre-training on large-scale datasets from the same domain to achieve competitive performance. In this work, we propose an alternative by introducing a new graph-based approach that models CT scans as structured graphs, leveraging axial slice triplets nodes processed through spectral domain convolution to enhance multi-label anomaly classification performance. Our method exhibits strong cross-dataset generalization, and competitive performance while achieving robustness to z-axis translation. An ablation study evaluates the contribution of each proposed component.

Keywords: 3D Medical Imaging · Chest Computed Tomography · Graph Neural Network · Spectral domain · Multi-label Anomaly Classification

1 Introduction

Computed Tomography (CT) is a fundamental modality in modern medical imaging, providing radiologists with detailed cross-sectional views of the human body to detect and characterize abnormalities. However, the increasing volume of CT scans has led to an important demand for automated deep learning-based methods to assist radiologists with their growing workload [6]. Deep learning has already demonstrated success in various CT-related tasks [1], including anomaly detection [16], organ segmentation [21], report generation [17], and synthetic volume reconstruction [16] for patient-specific modeling. Among these tasks, multi-label classification of anomalies in 3D CT volumes remains challenging due to the

N. Akash et al. (Eds.): EMERGE 2025 Workshops, LNCS 16534, pp. 47–57, 2026.
https://doi.org/10.1007/978-3-032-24182-5_5

computational complexity of processing volumetric data and the diverse range of pathological patterns. Early deep learning approaches leverage 3D Convolutional Neural Networks (CNNs), effectively capturing local spatial features but suffering from limited capabilities to model long-ranges dependencies [25]. More recently, Vision Transformers (ViTs) [12], initially designed for natural language processing [31], have been adapted to both 2D [15] and 3D [18] medical imaging. By enabling long-range spatial interactions through self-attention, ViTs have shown promise in various medical imaging tasks [3] through its capabilities to capture global information. However, they remain computationally expensive, requiring large-scale pretraining to generalize effectively [18]. Our work introduces CT-Graph, a new 2.5D GNN-based framework that models 3D chest CT scans as structured graphs, where each node represents a triplet of adjacent axial slices and edges are weighted by inter-slice spacing. This design enables efficient integration of local and global context while preserving spatial structure. Our approach offers the following key advantages:

- CT-Graph demonstrates strong cross-dataset generalization, maintaining consistent performance when trained on a public Turkish 3D chest CT dataset and evaluated on a separate dataset from the United States.
- Our edge weighting strategy based on z-axis distance spacing incorporates spatial awareness with no additional learnable parameters. Ablation studies confirm the effectiveness of GNN modules and graph connectivity patterns.
- By leveraging spectral domain convolution, CT-Graph improves anomaly classification performance and achieves robustness to z-axis translation.

2 Related Work

2.1 3D Visual Encoder

Feature aggregation in 3D medical imaging is crucial for balancing local and long-range dependencies while maintaining global spatial awareness. Early deep learning architectures primarily relied on 3D CNNs [1], which effectively capture local spatial dependencies. These models have been widely applied to tasks such as anomaly detection [20] and segmentation [28]. However, their intrinsic locality limits their ability to model long-range dependencies, which can be crucial for capturing global anatomical structures [25]. The self-attention mechanism [32], initially introduced for natural language processing tasks was rapidly adapted to the visual domain with ViTs [12]. The extension of ViTs [18] and Swin Transformers [34] to 3D tasks has shown promise in applications such as dense image captioning [9] and video processing [24]. In the context of CT imaging, GenerateCT leverages CT-ViT, inspired by ViViT [2], to integrate spatial and causal attention but requires extensive pretraining, limiting its practical applicability [18]. To mitigate computational challenges in 3D volume processing, CT-Net [13] proposes to group triplets of adjacent slices to replicate the three-channel structure of RGB images, extracting features using a pretrained 2D ResNet [19]. While CT-Net subsequently passes these representations through a lightweight

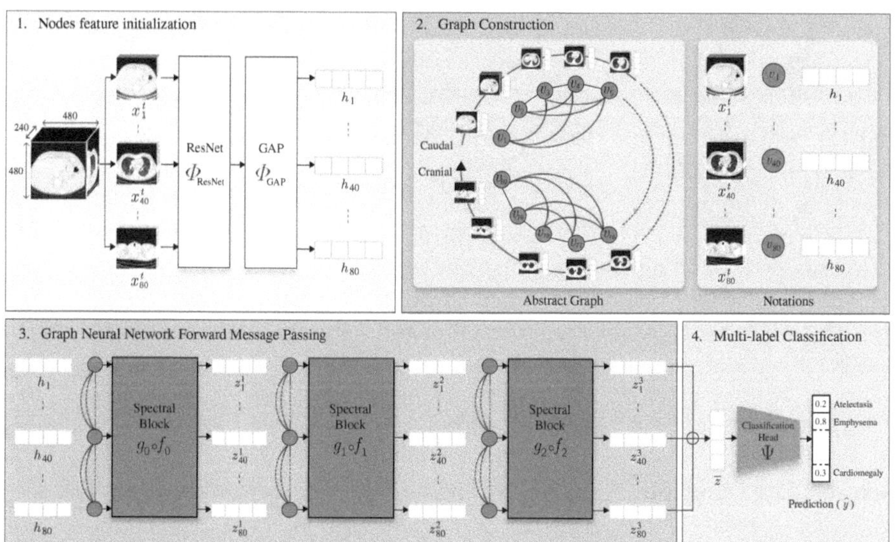

Fig. 1. CT-Graph introduces a structured graph-based architecture, where triplet axial slice features define nodes. Node interactions are modeled through spectral-domain convolutions, enabling contextual aggregation prior before classification.

3D CNN for dimensionality reduction, CT-Scroll [11] leverages an alternating global-local attention module to enable feature interactions, effectively reducing the number of parameters while improving classification performance.

2.2 Graph Neural Networks

In various application domains such as biology [29] or transportation [26], graphs are a common representation of data found in nature [33]. A graph, denoted as $\mathcal{G} = \{\mathcal{V}, \mathcal{E}\}$ consists of a set of edges $\mathcal{E}$ which model the connections between a set of nodes $\mathcal{V}$. In deep learning, GNNs have become the main approach for tasks involving graph-structured data [4], where each node is associated with a vector representation, which is iteratively updated through neighborhood aggregation during the forward message passing process. Representative models mainly include Convolutional GNNs, which aggregate neighboring node features through graph-based convolutions [10] or Attentional GNNs, which leverage attention mechanisms to weigh the importance of neighbors' contributions [7]. In medical imaging, GNNs have been used in tasks such as medical knowledge integration in radiology report generation [23] and Whole Slide Image analysis [14]. Specifically to 3D medical imaging, recent approaches have explored multi-view modeling, where each node encodes a triplet of orthogonal slices with axial, coronal, and sagittal views to capture complementary anatomical information [22].

3 Method

As shown in Fig. 1, CT-Graph models the 3D CT scan as a graph of *triplet axial CT slices* connected by their *physical z-axis distance*. Each node corresponds to a triplet of axial slices connected by neighborhood nodes with an edge weighted by their physical distance. Node features interact through a GNN module before being summed and given to a classification head.

Triplet Slices Feature Extraction. Following a strategy similar to CT-Net [13], we partition the input volume $x \in \mathbb{R}^{240\times480\times480}$ into non-overlapping triplets of slices, noted $\{x_i^t\}_{i=1}^{80}$ forming a tensor of dimension $80 \times 3 \times 480 \times 480$. Each triplet is processed by a ResNet [19] Φ_{ResNet} pretrained on ImageNet [30] to extract a corresponding feature map. The feature maps are then processed independently, with each one being passed through a Global Average Pooling (GAP) layer [11] Φ_{GAP} to obtain a compact vector representation for each triplet, noted $h_i \in \mathbb{R}^{512}$ ($i \in \{1, \dots, 80\}$), such that:

$$h_i = (\Phi_{\text{GAP}} \circ \Phi_{\text{ResNet}})(x_i^t), \quad \forall\, i \in \{1, \dots, 80\}. \tag{1}$$

Graph Construction. We define the volumetric representation as a graph $\mathcal{G} = (\mathcal{V}, \mathcal{E}, H, A)$, where:

- $\mathcal{V} = \{v_i\}_{i=1}^{N}$ is the set of nodes, where each node v_i represents a triplet of consecutive slices. Hence, the number of nodes is $N = 80$.
- $\mathcal{E} \subseteq \mathcal{V} \times \mathcal{V}$ is the set of edges, where an edge $(v_i, v_j) \in \mathcal{E}$ is weighted based on a function of inter-triplet distance and z-axis spacing. An undirected edge $(v_i, v_j) \in \mathcal{E}$ is established if and only if the corresponding triplet slices are separated by at most $q \in \mathbb{N}^+$ other triplet slices in the sequence, such that:

$$\mathcal{E} = \{(v_i, v_j) \mid |i - j| \leq q\}. \tag{2}$$

- $H = \{h_1, \dots, h_N\} \in \mathbb{R}^{N\times d}$ is the node feature matrix, where $\mathbf{h}_i \in \mathbb{R}^d$ denotes the feature embedding of node v_i ($\forall\, i \in \{1, \dots, N\}$). We set $d = 512$.
- $A \in \mathbb{R}^{N\times N}$ is the weighted adjacency matrix, where $A_{ij} = w_{i,j} \in \mathbb{R}^+$ encodes the connectivity and spatial relationship between triplets, $w_{i,j}$ being the edge weight such that:

$$A_{ij} = \begin{cases} w_{ij}, & \text{if } (v_i, v_j) \in \mathcal{E} \\ 0, & \text{otherwise.} \end{cases} \tag{3}$$

Graph Neural Network Module. A key challenge in this formulation is the variability in anatomical positioning across patients due to differences in scan length and body proportions. Traditional spatial graph convolutions, such as GraphConv [27], aggregate information from fixed local neighborhoods, which can be suboptimal in this context as anatomical structures do not consistently align across scans. Instead, we leverage Chebyshev convolutions [10] to define graph convolutions in the spectral domain, each followed by a feedforward neural network. Unlike spatial approaches, which struggle with non-uniform neighborhood structures [8], ChebConv utilizes polynomial approximations of the graph Laplacian [5] to capture hierarchical feature representations while preserving spatial localization. This allows the model to adapt to variations in caudal-cranial slice positioning and effectively learn long-range anatomical relationships, making it more robust to inter-patient variability. Our GNN module, denoted as Φ_{GNN}, consists of 3 Chebyshev Convolutional Layers [10], each noted f_n ($n \in \{0, 1, 2\}$) and followed by a feedforward neural network consisting of a linear layer followed by a ReLU, denoted as g_n, matching the depth of CT-Scroll [11] for fair comparison. For each layer, the scaled and normalized Laplacian $\hat{L}$ is defined as:

$$\hat{L} = \frac{2}{\lambda_{\max}}(D - A) - I\,, \tag{4}$$

where $\lambda_{\max}$ is the largest eigenvalue of the graph Laplacian $L = D - A$. The degree matrix D is a diagonal matrix where $D_{i,i} = \sum_{j=1}^{N} w_{i,j}$. $w_{i,j}$ denotes the edge weight from source node i to target node j, defined such that:

$$w_{i,j} = 1 + \frac{1}{1 + dist(i,j)} = 1 + \frac{1}{1 + 3 \times |i - j| \times s_z}\,, \tag{5}$$

where s_z is the spacing along the z-axis in decimetre. The convolution operation is parameterized using Chebyshev polynomials $T_j(\hat{L}) \in \mathbb{R}^{N \times N}$, resulting in a recurrence relation for the transformation of the node feature matrix. Let $Z^0 = H$ be the initial node feature matrix, $\theta_k \in \mathbb{R}^{d \times d}$ be the learnable parameters, and K be the Chebyshev filter size fixed to 3 for all experiments, to align with common practice [10]. The recurrence relation is given by:

$$Z^{n+1} = (g_n \circ f_n)(Z^n) = g_n(\sum_{k=0}^{K-1} T_k(\hat{L}) Z^n \theta_k), \quad \forall\, n \in \{0, 1, 2\}\,. \tag{6}$$

The GNN module Φ_{GNN} produces the final output vector representation, which we denote as $Z = Z^3 \in \mathbb{R}^{N \times d}$ and which is defined as:

$$Z = \{z_1^3, \ldots, z_N^3\} = \Phi_{\text{GNN}}(H)\,. \tag{7}$$

Feature Aggregation. The obtained vector representations are aggregated through summation to derive a vector representation, denoted as $\bar{z} \in \mathbb{R}^d$, which is subsequently passed to a classification head Ψ implemented as a lightweight multilayer perceptron. Ψ predicts the logit vector $\hat{y} \in \mathbb{R}^{18}$. The model is trained on a multi-label classification task using Binary Cross-Entropy as the loss function.

4 Experimental Results

4.1 Dataset Preparation

We train and evaluate our methods on the public CT-RATE dataset [16], which consists of non-contrast chest CT scans with 18 annotated anomalies extracted from radiology reports. The training set includes 17,799 unique patients, while

Table 1. Quantitative evaluation on the CT-RATE and Rad-ChestCT test sets. Reported mean and standard deviation metrics were computed over 5 independant runs. **Best** results are in bold, <u>second best</u> are underlined.

Dataset	Method	F1	Recall	AUROC	Accuracy
CT-RATE	Random Pred.	27.78 ±0.51	50.42 ±1.05	49.88 ±0.62	49.89 ±0.31
	ViViT [2]	49.91 ±0.28	66.39 ±1.48	79.19 ±0.28	75.95 ±0.71
	Swin3D [24]	50.64 ±0.25	<u>67.96</u> ±0.58	79.94 ±0.15	75.95 ±0.25
	CT-Net [13]	51.39 ±0.50	66.42 ±1.99	79.37 ±0.27	77.37 ±0.40
	CNN3D [1]	52.92 ±1.08	67.60 ±1.01	81.47 ±0.78	77.80 ±0.37
	CT-Scroll [11]	<u>53.97</u> ±0.21	65.36 ±1.91	<u>81.80</u> ±0.22	**79.49** ±0.45
	CT-Graph	**54.59** ±0.17	**68.77** ±0.92	**82.44** ±0.14	<u>78.66</u> ±0.36
Rad-ChestCT	Random Pred.	35.91 ±0.41	51.51 ±0.75	49.68 ±0.55	50.40 ±0.32
	ViViT [2]	48.59 ±0.97	69.27 ±1.64	67.83 ±0.38	60.22 ±1.15
	Swin3D [24]	47.98 ±0.41	66.76 ±0.63	67.29 ±0.23	60.67 ±0.60
	CT-Net [13]	47.53 ±0.93	68.45 ±1.18	67.71 ±0.83	60.05 ±1.93
	CNN3D [1]	<u>49.28</u> ±0.93	**70.47** ±0.73	71.13 ±0.62	61.08 ±0.60
	CT-Scroll [11]	48.55 ±0.54	66.63 ±1.49	<u>71.21</u> ±0.37	**63.02** ±0.93
	CT-Graph	**49.52** ±0.76	<u>69.30</u> ±1.48	**72.18** ±0.29	<u>62.60</u>±0.52

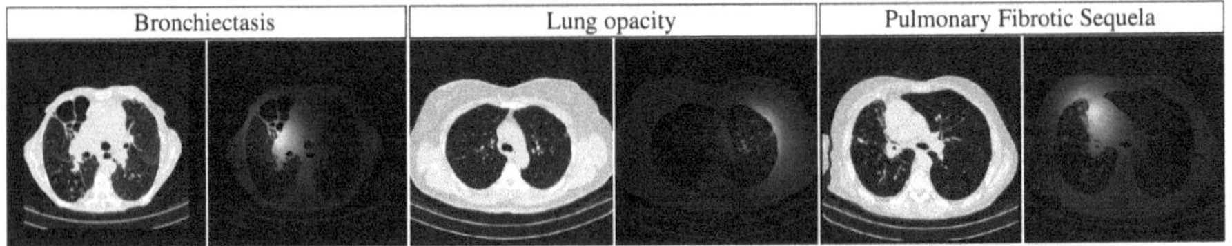

Fig. 2. GradCAM activation maps extracted from the 2D ResNet module.

the validation and test sets both contain 1,314 unique patients. Additionally, we extend our evaluation on the publicly available Rad-ChestCT dataset [13], comprising non-contrast chest CT scans from 1,344 unique patients, focusing on the 16 anomalies shared with CT-RATE [16]. Consistent with prior work [11, 17], volumes for both datasets are center-cropped or padded to a resolution of 240×480×480, with a spacing of 0.75 mm on the x and y and 1.5 mm on the z axis. Hounsfield Unit values are clipped to the range $[-1000, 200]$, reflecting practical diagnostic limits [17].

4.2 Implementation Details

CT-Graph and baseline methods are trained with a batch size of 4 using the AdamW optimizer with $(\beta_1, \beta_2) = (0.9, 0.99)$ and a weight decay of 0.01. The learning schedule follows a cosine decay with a warm-up phase of 20,000 steps, a maximum learning rate of 0.0001, and training runs for 200,000 iterations.

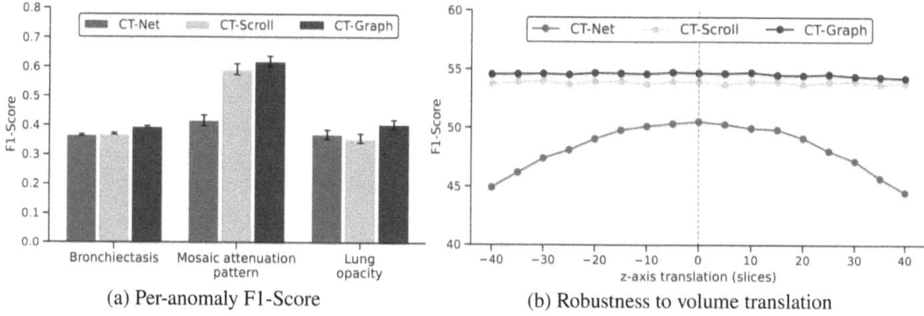

(a) Per-anomaly F1-Score (b) Robustness to volume translation

Fig. 3. (a) Per-anomaly F1 Score comparison for the 3 anomalies with highest improvement over baselines. (b) Model robustness to z-axis volume shift. F1 are reported for volumes translated along the z-axis with minimum-value padding.

4.3 Quantitative Results

For each method and each label, we select the threshold that maximizes F1-Score on the validation set and report all metrics on the test set. We compare our method against a 3D CNN, ViViT [2], a video-adapted Vision Transformer which also forms the architectural basis for CT-ViT, and Swin3D [34], an extension of Swin Transformer for volumetric data. We also include CT-Net [13] and CT-Scroll [11], two 2.5D approaches that employ CNN-based feature extractors. CT-Net relies on convolutional layers for feature aggregation and dimensionality reduction, whereas CT-Scroll leverages an alternating attention mechanism to capture cross-slice dependencies. ResNet-based models used ImageNet pretrained weights; others were initialized via weight inflation [35] for comparability. Table 1 shows that CT-Graph consistently outperforms all baselines across AUROC, F1-Score and Recall. On the `CT-RATE` test set, our method achieves an F1-Score of 54.59, representing a $+\Delta 1.15\%$ improvement over CT-Scroll [11] and $+\Delta 5.93\%$ over CT-Net [13]. For the F1-Score, a paired t-test comparing the performance of CT-Graph against each baseline consistently yields a p-value < 0.01, demonstrating statistical significance. As shown in Fig. 3a, CT-Graph yields the largest improvements on diffuse anomalies such as bronchiectasis, mosaic attenuation, and lung opacity. Reffering to Fig. 3b, both attention and spectral convolution demonstrate robustness to z-axis translations, whereas standard convolution is sensitive to such shifts. To evaluate this property, we simulate patient body shifts by applying controlled translations along the z-axis with appropriate padding. Figure 2 illustrates CT-Graph's ability to classify anomalies from relevent regions.

4.4 Ablation Study

Comparison of Representative GNNs. Table 2 highlights the performance gains achieved by incorporating Chebyshev Convolutions [10] in our GNN module. Compared to a direct neighborhood aggregation approach [27], ChebConv

Table 2. Comparison of graph connectivity schemes and GNN modules, evaluated on the CT-RATE test set. The neighborhood size is fixed to 16 for these runs.

Connectivity	Module	F1	AUROC	Accuracy
Fully connected	GATv2Conv [7]	53.72 ±0.34	81.56±0.03	78.04 ±0.31
	GraphConv [27]	53.73 ±0.36	81.99 ±0.40	78.15 ±0.31
	ChebConv [10]	54.40 ±0.15	82.34 ±0.12	79.01 ±0.55
Neighbourhood	GATv2Conv [7]	54.06 ±0.19	82.22 ±0.05	78.59 ±0.25
	GraphConv [27]	54.16 ±0.24	82.33 ±0.18	78.68 ±0.52
	ChebConv [10]	**54.41** ±0.12	**82.47** ±0.26	**79.12** ±0.53

Table 3. Impact of the neighbourhood size, using GraphConv. Neighborhood size, noted as q, refers to the number of nodes each node is connected to.

Neighbourhood size	F1 Score	Recall	Precision	AUROC	Accuracy
4	53.76 ±0.24	66.02 ±0.92	**47.84** ±0.22	82.22 ±0.05	**78.97** ±0.58
16	**54.14** ±0.24	67.99 ±0.75	47.34 ±0.30	**82.33** ±0.18	78.68 ±0.52
80 (Fully connected)	53.73 ±0.36	**69.34** ±0.91	45.80 ±0.59	81.99 ±0.40	78.15 ±0.31

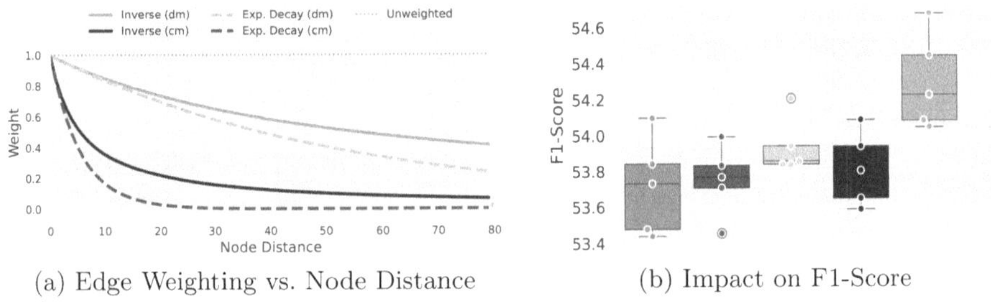

(a) Edge Weighting vs. Node Distance (b) Impact on F1-Score

Fig. 4. Impact of the edge weighting functions, on the CT-RATE test set. We use a GraphConv module and a fully connected graph for all experiments.

improves AUROC by $+\Delta 0.42\%$ and F1-Score by $+\Delta 1.25\%$, suggesting that spectral-domain convolutions may enhance feature aggregation while demonstrating robustness to variations in cranial-caudal slice positioning (Fig. 3). Inference time takes approximately 70 milliseconds for all GNN variants.

Graph Construction. Table 2 and Table 3 demonstrate that neighborhood graph construction consistently improves AUROC and F1-score across all GNN variants, with particularly pronounced gains for GATv2Conv and GraphConv, with ChebConv showing marginal gains.

Impact of the Weight Function. Among the evaluated edge weighting functions, the inverse function (see Eq. 5) with z-axis spacing measured in decimeters (dm) yields the best classification performance, as illustrated in Fig. 4.

5 Discussion and Conclusion

In this work, we introduced CT-Graph, a new graph-based approach for multi-label anomaly classification from 3D Chest CT volumes. Each scan is represented as a structured graph, where nodes correspond to triplets of adjacent axial slices. To enable effective feature aggregation across this graph, we leverage a spectral approach based on Chebyshev convolution, which captures both short-range and long-range dependencies along the axial direction. Additionally, we show that incorporating spatially-aware graph structures, through both weighted edges and constrained neighborhood connectivity, enhances performance across multiple Graph Neural Network variants. CT-Graph demonstrates robustness to variations in patient body positioning along the z-axis and provides a flexible framework for modeling volumetric data. Future work may include anatomical segmentation-driven graph construction, transformer-based hybridization with patch representations, multi-view modeling extension, and exploration of architectural factors such as convolution depth and Chebyshev filter size.

Disclosure of Interests. The authors have no competing interests to declare that are relevant to the content of this article.

References

1. Anaya-Isaza, A., Mera-Jiménez, L., Zequera-Diaz, M.: An overview of deep learning in medical imaging. Inform. Med. Unlocked **26**, 100723 (2021)
2. Arnab, A., Dehghani, M., Heigold, G., Sun, C., Lucic, M., Schmid, C.: ViViT: a video vision transformer. In: 2021 IEEE/CVF International Conference on Computer Vision (ICCV), Montreal, QC, Canada, pp. 6816–6826. IEEE (2021)
3. Azad, R., et al.: Advances in medical image analysis with vision Transformers: a comprehensive review. Med. Image Anal. **91**, 103000 (2024)
4. Bechler-Speicher, M., Globerson, A., Gilad-Bachrach, R.: The intelligible and effective graph neural additive networks (2024). arXiv:2406.01317 [cs]
5. Belkin, M., Niyogi, P.: Laplacian eigenmaps and spectral techniques for embedding and clustering. In: Advances in Neural Information Processing Systems, vol. 14. MIT Press (2001)
6. Broder, J., Warshauer, D.M.: Increasing utilization of computed tomography in the adult emergency department, 2000–2005. Emerg. Radiol. **13**(1), 25–30 (2006)
7. Brody, S., Alon, U., Yahav, E.: How attentive are graph attention networks? (2022). arXiv:2105.14491 [cs]
8. Bruna, J., Zaremba, W., Szlam, A., LeCun, Y.: Spectral networks and locally connected networks on graphs (2014). arXiv:1312.6203 [cs]
9. Chen, D.Z., Hu, R., Chen, X., Nießner, M., Chang, A.X.: UniT3D: a unified transformer for 3D dense captioning and visual grounding (2022). arXiv:2212.00836 [cs]

10. Defferrard, M., Bresson, X., Vandergheynst, P.: Convolutional neural networks on graphs with fast localized spectral filtering (2017). arXiv:1606.09375 [cs]
11. Di Piazza, T., Lazarus, C., Nempont, O., Boussel, L.: Imitating radiological scrolling: a global-local attention model for 3D chest CT volumes multi-label anomaly classification (2025)
12. Dosovitskiy, A., et al.: An image is worth 16 × 16 words: transformers for image recognition at scale (2021). arXiv:2010.11929 [cs]
13. Draelos, R.L., et al.: Machine-learning-based multiple abnormality prediction with large-scale chest computed tomography volumes. Med. Image Anal. **67**, 101857 (2021)
14. Guo, Z., Zhao, W., Wang, S., Yu, L.: HIGT: hierarchical interaction graph-transformer for whole slide image analysis (2023). arXiv:2309.07400 [cs]
15. Halder, A., Gharami, S., Sadhu, P., Singh, P.K., Woźniak, M., Ijaz, M.F.: Implementing vision transformer for classifying 2D biomedical images. Sci. Rep. **14**(1), 12567 (2024)
16. Hamamci, I.E., et al.: A foundation model utilizing chest CT volumes and radiology reports for supervised-level zero-shot detection of abnormalities (2024). arXiv:2403.17834 [cs]
17. Hamamci, I.E., Er, S., Menze, B.: CT2Rep: automated radiology report generation for 3D medical imaging (2024). arXiv:2403.06801 [cs, eess]
18. Hamamci, I.E., et al.: GenerateCT: text-conditional generation of 3D chest CT volumes (2023). arXiv:2305.16037 [cs]
19. He, K., Zhang, X., Ren, S., Sun, J.: Deep Residual learning for image recognition (2015). arXiv:1512.03385 [cs]
20. Ibrahim, D.M., Elshennawy, N.M., Sarhan, A.M.: Deep-chest: multi-classification deep learning model for diagnosing COVID-19, pneumonia, and lung cancer chest diseases. Comput. Biol. Med. **132**, 104348 (2021)
21. Ilesanmi, A.E., Ilesanmi, T.O., Ajayi, B.O.: Reviewing 3D convolutional neural network approaches for medical image segmentation. Heliyon **10**(6), e27398 (2024)
22. Kiechle, J., Lang, D.M., Fischer, S.M., Felsner, L., Peeken, J.C., Schnabel, J.A.: Graph neural networks: a suitable alternative to MLPs in latent 3D medical image classification? (2024). arXiv:2407.17219 [cs]
23. Liu, F., Wu, X., Ge, S., Fan, W., Zou, Y.: Exploring and distilling posterior and prior knowledge for radiology report generation (2021). arXiv:2106.06963 [cs]
24. Liu, Z., et al.: Video Swin Transformer (2021). arXiv:2106.13230 [cs]
25. Ma, J., Li, F., Wang, B.: U-mamba: enhancing long-range dependency for biomedical image segmentation (2024). arXiv:2401.04722 [eess]
26. Makarov, N., Narayanan, S., Antoniou, C.: Graph neural network surrogate for strategic transport planning (2024). arXiv:2408.07726 [cs]
27. Morris, C., et al.: Weisfeiler and Leman go neural: higher-order graph neural networks (2021). arXiv:1810.02244 [cs]
28. Rayed, M.E., Islam, S.M.S., Niha, S.I., Jim, J.R., Kabir, M.M., Mridha, M.F.: Deep learning for medical image segmentation: state-of-the-art advancements and challenges. Inform. Med. Unlocked **47**, 101504 (2024)
29. Reiser, P., et al.: Graph neural networks for materials science and chemistry. Commun. Mater. **3**(1), 1–18 (2022)
30. Russakovsky, O., et al.: ImageNet large scale visual recognition challenge (2015). arXiv:1409.0575 [cs]
31. Tucudean, G., Bucos, M., Dragulescu, B., Caleanu, C.D.: Natural language processing with transformers: a review. PeerJ. Comput. Sci. **10**, e2222 (2024)

32. Vaswani, A., et al.: Attention is all you need (2023). arXiv:1706.03762 [cs]
33. Veličković, P.: Everything is connected: graph neural networks. Curr. Opin. Struct. Biol. **79**, 102538 (2023). arXiv:2301.08210 [cs]
34. Yang, Y.Q., et al.: Swin3D: a pretrained transformer backbone for 3D indoor scene understanding (2023). arXiv:2304.06906 [cs]
35. Zhang, Y., Huang, S.C., Zhou, Z., Lungren, M.P., Yeung, S.: Adapting pre-trained vision transformers from 2D to 3D through weight inflation improves medical image segmentation (2023). arXiv:2302.04303 [cs]

Automated Method Design for Cancer Image Classification by Differential Evolution and Ensembling

Natalia Oviedo Acosta[1,2](✉), Stefan Klein[1], and Martijn P. A. Starmans[1,2]

[1] Department of Radiology and Nuclear Medicine, Erasmus MC, Rotterdam, The Netherlands
{s.klein,m.starmans}@erasmusmc.nl
n.oviedoacosta@erasmusmc.nl, s.klein@erasmusmc.nl, m.starmans@erasmusmc.nl
[2] Department of Pathology, Erasmus MC, Rotterdam, The Netherlands
n.oviedoacosta@erasmusmc.nl

Abstract. Developing deep learning models for cancer image classification requires many method design choices, such as in data preprocessing, model architecture, hyperparameters and training procedures. Typically, these are manually tuned, a process that is time-consuming, expert-dependent, and often irreproducible. To address these challenges, we propose an automated machine learning (AutoML) framework that optimizes model design without human intervention. To ensure a comprehensive exploration of diverse architectures and hyperparameter configurations, we define a search space based on state-of-the-art literature in cancer imaging. Our framework employs Differential Evolution and Hyperband (DEHB), which integrates evolutionary search algorithms to balance search space exploration and exploitation, combined with adaptive resource allocation to mitigate the high computational cost of training multiple models. To enhance model robustness and reduce overfitting in data-limited scenarios, we incorporate ensembling. We validate our approach on four public cancer classification datasets encompassing 750 patients with either MRI or CT. The proposed framework demonstrates higher performance when compared to a DenseNet-121 baseline. While exploring multiple configurations, our approach reduces training time by a factor of two to five compared to the baseline. By automating model design and improving generalization across datasets, our framework has substantial potential for broad applications across cancer imaging, thereby streamlining deep learning model development.

Keywords: AutoML · evolutionary algorithms · hyperparameter optimization · computer-aided diagnosis

1 Introduction

Deep learning has substantially advanced cancer image analysis by enabling precise and early diagnosis through AI-driven models [17]. However, developing

N. Akash et al. (Eds.): EMERGE 2025 Workshops, LNCS 16534, pp. 58–67, 2026.
https://doi.org/10.1007/978-3-032-24182-5_6

these models remains a labor-intensive process that requires numerous decisions regarding data preprocessing, model architecture, hyperparameters, and model training. Commonly the majority of these choices are made manually through a heuristic trial-and-error process, which is time-consuming, prone to overfitting [10], limits reproducibility [12,21], may lead to suboptimal solutions [12] and can be resource-intensive, making it inefficient [16,24].

Among cancer imaging tasks, classification poses unique challenges, as it often relies on a limited number of image-level labels, leading to small and heterogeneous datasets that make model development highly sensitive to hyperparameter choices and prone to overfitting, where models may learn spurious correlations instead of generalizable patterns [25]. To address these challenges, we propose an automated method design framework based on Automated Machine Learning (AutoML) [12] to streamline and optimize deep learning model development for cancer image classification. AutoML has been gaining significant traction in recent years and is increasingly being adopted in medical imaging. Promising results have been reported in both segmentation [4] and classification tasks [7], with several recent studies providing comprehensive reviews and benchmarks tailored to clinical applications [2,14]. As a next step in this direction, our framework automates key design decisions, including data preprocessing, model selection, hyperparameter tuning, and model training, thereby eliminating manual intervention. We leverage Differential Evolution and Hyperband (DEHB) [3], a state-of-the-art AutoML optimization algorithm, to efficiently explore large hyperparameter spaces and improve both convergence speed and model performance. We hypothesize that integrating DEHB into the model development pipeline will substantially accelerate training compared to manual tuning. Additionally, we incorporate ensembling strategies to regularize DEHB optimization and improve overall performance.

2 Methods

To automate model design, given a training dataset D_{train} and a validation dataset D_{val}, we define an optimization function with the objective of identifying the optimal hyperparameter configuration x^* that minimizes the average validation loss $\mathcal{L}$ over K_{training} iterations (e.g., cross-validation). We formulate the optimization of any method design choice, including data preprocessing, model architecture, and model training, as a combined method selection and hyperparameter optimization problem. Formally, we express this as follows:

$$x^* = \arg\min_{x \in X} \frac{1}{K_{\text{training}}} \sum_{k=1}^{K_{\text{training}}} \mathcal{L}(x, D_{\text{train},k}, D_{\text{val},k}, b), \tag{1}$$

where x represents a hyperparameter configuration, X denotes the hyperparameter search space, and a given computational budget b (i.e., number of epochs).

Manual tuning and conventional tuning strategies such as exhaustive grid search or random search over X are computationally expensive, as these methods lack efficient resource allocation mechanisms. To address this, we propose to employ DEHB, which effectively balances the exploration of the search space with a focus on promising solutions through an evolutionary algorithm, while efficiently managing computational resources using Hyperband [16]. By leveraging Differential Evolution (DE) [18] for guided search and Hyperband for adaptive resource allocation, DEHB provides a more efficient and scalable approach to hyperparameter optimization, making it particularly well-suited for large and complex search spaces as well as resource-intensive model training.

2.1 Differential Evolution and Hyperband (DEHB)

As presented in Algorithm 1, DEHB is initialized by evaluating a population of Q candidates, i.e., set configurations of hyperparameters randomly sampled from X. Initially, each configuration is trained on the minimum budget b_{min}, and its validation loss $\mathcal{L}(x, D_{\text{train}}, D_{\text{val}}, b_{\text{min}})$ is measured. After initialization, Hyperband dynamically allocates computational resources by discarding poorly performing configurations through successive halving. Configurations are evaluated in progressive stages, where in each stage only the top $1/\eta$ fraction of candidates continues to the next stage with an increased budget b, while the rest are eliminated. The selection is based solely on the validation loss observed at the current budget level, without the use of any patience mechanism. Parameter η, known as the aggressiveness factor, controls how many configurations are discarded. The number of remaining candidates at stage s is therefore $Q \cdot (1/\eta)^s$, making the reduction schedule deterministic. The budget b increases at each stage according to the Hyperband schedule, typically growing multiplicatively with η. This process iterates until a predefined b_{max} is reached or only one configuration remains. Once Hyperband has selected the top-performing candidates for further evaluation, DEHB extends this process by continuing the search with evolutionary steps. The general procedure stops once all P configurations have been evaluated and the x^* is selected based on the validation loss.

Mutation. Each configuration x_i represents a vector of chosen hyperparameters. New candidate configurations, or mutant vectors v_i, are generated through a mutation process that introduces controlled variations based on existing ones. Specifically, mutation is performed as follows:

$$v_i = x_r + F \cdot (x_a - x_b),$$

where x_r, x_a, x_b are randomly selected hyperparameter configurations from the population, and F is a scaling factor controlling the magnitude of change within the range (0,1].

Crossover. After mutation, a new candidate vector u_i is generated through crossover, where each parameter is inherited from the original vector x_i or the mutant vector v_i. Each configuration vector (e.g., x_i) consists of N hyperparameters, denoted as x_i^j, v_i^j, and u_i^j, where $j \in \{1, 2, \ldots, N\}$ indexes the individual

Algorithm 1 Differential Evolution and Hyperband (DEHB)

Require: Search space $\mathcal{X}$, budgets $b_{\min}$, $b_{\max}$, reduction factor η, max evaluations P

Randomly sample Q configurations from $\mathcal{X}$ into $P_{b_{\min}}$
Evaluate all configurations in $P_{b_{\min}}$ at budget $b_{\min}$
while total function evaluations $< P$ **do**
  for each budget b in $\{b_{\min}, \eta b_{\min}, \eta^2 b_{\min}, \ldots, b_{\max}\}$ **do**
    Select top $1/\eta$ fraction of configurations from previous budget as parent pool
    for each configuration x_i in the parent pool **do**
      Generate mutant vector v_i
      Generate trial vector u_i via crossover between x_i and v_i
      Evaluate u_i on budget b
      Replace x_i in the population if u_i performs better
    end for
  end for
end while
return x^*: best configuration across all budgets

hyperparameters. Crossover is performed independently for each hyperparameter j, selecting between v_i^j and x_i^j according to the following rule:

$$u_i^j = \begin{cases} v_i^j, & \text{if } (z \sim \mathcal{U}(0,1)) \leq Cr \text{ or } (j = j_{\text{rand}}) \\ x_i^j, & \text{otherwise} \end{cases}$$

where Cr is the crossover probability, determining the likelihood of inheriting parameters from v_i. The index j_{rand}, randomly selected from $\{1, 2, \ldots, N\}$, ensures that at least one parameter comes from v_i, to prevent $u_i = x_i$. This process allows crossover to integrate information from the mutant vector while preserving useful characteristics from the original configuration.

Selection. The selection process then compares the performance of u_i against its corresponding parent configuration x_i using the optimization function in Eq. 1. If u_i achieves a lower validation loss than x_i, it replaces x_i in the population for the next iteration. Otherwise, x_i is retained.

2.2 Search Space

The performance of an AutoML framework highly depends on the search space, i.e., the potential hyperparameter configurations. Since non-architectural design choices such as data preprocessing, augmentation, model selection, and model training can be equally important as architectural ones [6,13], we construct a comprehensive search space covering all these aspects, including discrete and categorical hyperparameters, which motivates our choice of DEHB as the optimization strategy. To reduce computational burden, we set a GPU memory constraint to filter out infeasible configurations and maintain efficient training times. The complete search space is illustrated in Fig. 1.

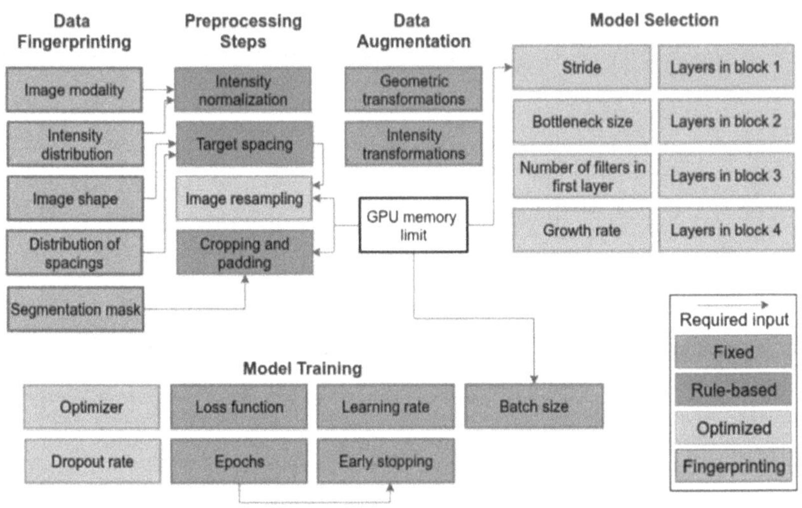

Design choice	Configuration
Intensity normalization	MRI: per-image z-score normalization. CT: global percentile clipping followed by z-score normalization.
Target spacing	Median, mean, fixed isotropic (1×1×1 mm), and isotropic based on the median volume.
Cropping and padding	Crop the bounding box if its dimensions exceed available memory, and pad if any dimension is below the model's minimum size.
Image resampling	Linear interpolation
Optimizer	SGD with Nesterov momentum (μ = 0.99), Adam or Adadelta
Dropout rate	{**0.0**, 0.1, 0.2, 0.3, 0.4, 0.5}
Bottleneck size	{1, 2, **4**}
Number of layers in the first layer	{12, 32, **64**}

Design choice	Configuration
Growth rates	{12, 16, 20, 26, **32**}
Layers in block 1	{4, **6**, 8, 10}
Layers in block 2	{8, **12**, 16, 20}
Layers in block 3	{16, **24**, 32, 40}
Layers in block 4	{8, 12, **16**, 20}
Stride	{1, **2**, 3}
Data augmentation	Flipping, rotations, zooming, scaling, and adjusting contrast
Loss function	Cross-entropy loss
Learning rate	ExponentialLR scheduler that decays the learning rate by a factor of 0.9
Epochs	Min: 30, Max: 50
Batch size	Batch size 1 and gradient accumulation after 5 epochs.
Early stopping	40% of the number of epochs

Fig. 1. Overview of the proposed search space for cancer image classification. Default values are shown in bold.

Inspired by nnU-Net [13], we introduce dataset fingerprinting to extract key information about the input data, including modality, intensity distribution, image shape, and spacing. These properties are used to define rule-based constraints that both filter infeasible configurations and determine default hyper-parameter values within our AutoML search space.

Preprocessing includes intensity normalization and resampling. To account for differences in resolution due to scanner variations, we included different target spacings. For cropping and padding, we constrained the image sizes to a maximum of 512 voxels in all three dimensions. As our datasets contain the tumor segmentation masks, we applied tumor-centered cropping to focus on the region of interest while reducing unnecessary background. To prevent test-time bias, we applied all preprocessing steps described above exclusively to the training data.

The backbone architecture used is DenseNet [11], which has demonstrated strong performance in cancer imaging tasks due to its efficient feature propagation and parameter efficiency, making it suitable for learning from limited and heterogeneous datasets [26]. Search ranges for bottleneck size, growth rate, initial filter count, and block depth were defined based on default DenseNet-121 values [11] and expanded to explore broader architectural variations.

For training parameters, the loss function was fixed to cross-entropy loss, a standard choice for classification tasks as stated in [19]. The learning rate is fixed, as prior work has shown that optimizing it can be unreliable under multi-fidelity optimization frameworks like Hyperband [15]. To ensure stable optimization with a batch size of one, gradient accumulation was combined with instance normalization to maintain consistent updates and training dynamics.

2.3 Ensembling

While DEHB aims to identify a single optimal configuration, the optimization landscape in medical imaging–particularly with small, heterogeneous datasets–can be noisy [8,17], and AutoML methods such as DEHB are prone to overfitting on the validation dataset [1]. To mitigate this and improve generalization, we construct ensembles by averaging predictions from multiple models trained with diverse configurations selected by DEHB, ensuring that only competitive candidates contribute while maintaining diversity across method design choices. Given a set of M selected hyperparameter configurations $\{x_1, \ldots, x_M\}$, each of which is evaluated across K different data splits (e.g., cross-validation folds), we obtain a total of $M \cdot K$ trained models.

The ensemble prediction $\hat{y}$ for an input z is computed as

$$\hat{y} = \frac{1}{M \cdot K} \sum_{m=1}^{M} \sum_{k=1}^{K} \hat{y}_{m,k}(z),$$

where $\hat{y}_{m,k}(z)$ denotes the prediction made by the model trained with configuration x_m on fold k. This formulation allows for flexibility in ensemble design: setting $M = 1$ yields an ensemble over data splits, while increasing M incorporates configuration-level diversity.

3 Experiments and Results

3.1 Dataset

For this study, four datasets from the publicly available WORC Database [23] are used, comprising 750 anonymized patients with various tumor types. Each dataset includes an MRI or CT scan, a tumor segmentation, and a tumor type label serving as the prediction target. The datasets contain 115 patients with liposarcoma or lipoma (Lipo), 203 with desmoid-type fibromatosis or extremity soft-tissue sarcomas (Desmoid), 186 with primary solid liver tumors (Liver), and 246 with gastrointestinal stromal tumors or similar intra-abdominal tumors (GIST).

3.2 Experimental Setup

To evaluate the framework, two baselines were used: (1) the WORC framework [22], previously validated on these datasets, and (2) DenseNet-121 [11] without hyperparameter tuning, trained from scratch for 100 epochs with 5-fold cross-validation using default settings.

For DEHB, the maximum and minimum fidelity levels (number of epochs) were set to $b_{\max} = 50$ and $b_{\min} = 30$, respectively. Other parameters followed default values [3]: $\eta = 2$, $F = 0.5$. Each dataset was split into 80% training and 20% test sets. All model selection and cross-validation procedures, including those for DEHB and DenseNet-121, were conducted within the training set using 5-fold cross-validation. DEHB performed $P = 10$ function evaluations per fold, selecting one best configuration per fold. These five configurations were retrained and evaluated across all five folds to obtain robust performance estimates, yielding 25 trained models per dataset. All experiments were run on 8×NVIDIA A40 48 GB GPUs using MONAI [5] for efficient medical image processing.

Model performance was primarily measured using ROC-AUC [9]. DEHB was evaluated in three ways: (1) the best configuration (lowest average validation loss across five folds) was retrained on the full 80% training set and tested on the 20% holdout; (2) a 5-Model Ensemble (5ME) was created by training the top configuration across all five folds ($M = 1$, $K = 5$); and (3) a 25-Model Ensemble (25ME), where the top five configurations were retrained across five folds ($M = 5$, $K = 5$), and their predictions averaged.

Computation Time. Wall-clock time was measured for each dataset to assess the efficiency of our framework, using $P = 50$ configurations. For the DenseNet-121 baseline, training was performed with default settings using a single configuration for 100 epochs. Since training all P configurations individually for the baseline would be computationally intensive, we estimated the cost by training once on the larger datasets (Desmoid and GIST) and averaging five runs on the smaller ones (Lipo and Liver). This simulation was intended to approximate the total wall-clock time that would be required if 50 different configurations, equivalent to those evaluated by DEHB, were trained from scratch using the DenseNet-121 baseline, enabling a fair comparison of computational cost.

3.3 Results

Table 1 compares the performance of different methods across all four datasets. The DEHB framework alone slightly underperforms both baselines on most datasets. However, incorporating the 5ME strategy with DEHB improves performance across most datasets, with a higher performance increase observed with DEHB + 25ME in all datasets.

Table 1. ROC-AUC for the four datasets, evaluated under three different setups: (1) WORC in 100× random-split cross-validation, (2) DenseNet-121 in 5-fold cross-validation, and (3) DEHB using a fixed 80/20 train/test split. The second row indicates the number of samples (N_s) for each dataset.

Model	Lipo	Liver	Desmoid	GIST
N_s	115	186	203	246
Baselines				
WORC	0.83	0.80	0.82	0.77
DenseNet-121	0.82	**0.88**	0.80	0.61
Framework				
DEHB	0.78	0.83	0.73	0.73
DEHB + 5ME	0.83	0.86	0.80	0.78
DEHB + 25ME	**0.87**	0.87	**0.83**	**0.81**

Computation Time. Our framework showed substantially lower computational cost across all datasets compared to the simulated 50x DenseNet-121 baseline. On Lipo, DEHB completed all $P = 50$ configurations in 95 h versus 650 for the baseline. For Liver, DEHB required 220 h (vs. 900), and for Desmoid, 340 h (vs. 1100). On GIST, the largest dataset, DEHB finished in 216 h (9 days), while the baseline was projected to take 3600 h (150 days). These results demonstrate a 2–5x speedup, indicating that the framework scales efficiently and enables automated model design without compromising runtime feasibility.

4 Discussion and Conclusion

This study presents an AutoML framework for cancer image classification that combines DEHB with ensembling for automated method design. DEHB identified multiple high-performing models with similar validation performance, as observed in five-fold cross-validation. Instead of relying solely on a single configuration, we aggregate these diverse models through ensembling to enhance robustness and generalization. Ensembling helps counteract overfitting by averaging individual model biases. Although the improvement varies across datasets, our results show that ensembles consistently match or outperform both the best individual DEHB model and the baselines in the majority of cases, supporting their complementary role. Moreover, DEHB substantially reduced computational time compared to the baseline by leveraging adaptive resource allocation, avoiding exhaustive training and minimizing the need for manual tuning. Further efficiency gains may be possible through techniques like reduced precision computations [20]. While our evaluation offers a practical comparison basis, the fixed 80/20 train/test split used for DEHB may limit comparability with baselines trained under different protocols. Future work will focus on aligning evaluation strategies. Additionally, although DenseNet-121 was used as the backbone, extending the framework to other architectures could offer broader insight into DEHB's generalizability.

Our results highlight the effectiveness of combining DEHB with ensembling to achieve competitive performance while significantly reducing computational cost. By efficiently exploring configurations across preprocessing, architecture, and training, the framework enables fully automated model design. This not only accelerates development but also improves reproducibility, reduces overfitting, and avoids suboptimal choices. These strengths make DEHB a compelling solution for optimizing deep learning in cancer imaging, especially in resource-constrained settings, and support more scalable, reproducible AI-driven diagnostics.

Acknowledgments. This work is part of the AIID project, funded by the Dutch Research Council (NWO) under the AiNed Fellowship Grants programme (project number NGF. 1607.22.025).

Disclosure of Interests. The authors have no competing interests to declare that are relevant to the content of this article.

References

1. Al-Helali, B., Chen, Q., Xue, B., Zhang, M.: Multi-tree genetic programming for feature construction-based domain adaptation in symbolic regression with incomplete data. In: Proceedings of the 2020 Genetic and Evolutionary Computation Conference, pp. 913–921 (2020)
2. Ali, M.J., Essaid, M., Moalic, L., Idoumghar, L.: A review of automl optimization techniques for medical image applications. Comput. Med. Imaging Graph. **118**, 102441 (2024)
3. Awad, N., Mallik, N., Hutter, F.: DEHB: evolutionary hyperband for scalable, robust and efficient hyperparameter optimization. arXiv preprint arXiv:2105.09821 (2021)
4. Becktepe, J., Hennig, L., Oeltze-Jafra, S., Lindauer, M.: Auto-nnU-Net: towards automated medical image segmentation. arXiv preprint arXiv:2505.16561 (2025)
5. Cardoso, M.J., et al.: Monai: an open-source framework for deep learning in healthcare. arXiv preprint arXiv:2211.02701 (2022)
6. De Raad, K., et al.: The effect of preprocessing on convolutional neural networks for medical image segmentation. In: 2021 IEEE 18th International Symposium on Biomedical Imaging (ISBI), pp. 655–658. IEEE (2021)
7. Elangovan, K., Lim, G., Ting, D.: A comparative study of an on premise automl solution for medical image classification. Sci. Rep. **14**(1), 10483 (2024)
8. Esteva, A., et al.: A guide to deep learning in healthcare. Nat. Med. **25**(1), 24–29 (2019)

9. Fawcett, T.: ROC graphs: notes and practical considerations for researchers. Mach. Learn. **31**(1), 1–38 (2004)
10. Hosseini, M., Powell, M., Collins, J., Callahan-Flintoft, C., Jones, W., Bowman, H., Wyble, B.: I tried a bunch of things: the dangers of unexpected overfitting in classification of brain data. Neurosci. Biobehav. Rev. **119**, 456–467 (2020)
11. Huang, G., Liu, Z., Van Der Maaten, L., Weinberger, K.Q.: Densely connected convolutional networks. In: Proceedings of the IEEE Conference on Computer Vision and Pattern Recognition, pp. 4700–4708 (2017)
12. Hutter, F., Kotthoff, L., Vanschoren, J.: Automated Machine Learning: Methods, Systems, Challenges. Springer, Cham (2019)
13. Isensee, F., Jaeger, P.F., Kohl, S.A., Petersen, J., Maier-Hein, K.H.: nnU-Net: a self-configuring method for deep learning-based biomedical image segmentation. Nat. Methods **18**(2), 203–211 (2021)
14. Jidney, T.T., et al.: AutoML systems for medical imaging. In: Data driven approaches on medical imaging, pp. 91–106. Springer, Cham (2023)
15. Lee, H., Lee, G., Kim, J., Cho, S., Kim, D., Yoo, D.: Improving multi-fidelity optimization with a recurring learning rate for hyperparameter tuning. In: Proceedings of the IEEE/CVF Winter Conference on Applications of Computer Vision, pp. 2309–2318 (2023)
16. Li, L., Jamieson, K., DeSalvo, G., Rostamizadeh, A., Talwalkar, A.: Hyperband: a novel bandit-based approach to hyperparameter optimization. J. Mach. Learn. Res. **18**(185), 1–52 (2018)
17. Litjens, G., et al.: A survey on deep learning in medical image analysis. Med. Image Anal. **42**, 60–88 (2017)
18. Price, K.V., Storn, R.M., Lampinen, J.A.: Differential Evolution: A Practical Approach to Global Optimization. Springer, Cham (2005)
19. Rajaraman, S., Zamzmi, G., Antani, S.K.: Novel loss functions for ensemble-based medical image classification. PLoS ONE **16**(12), e0261307 (2021)
20. Selvan, R., Schön, J., Dam, E.B.: Operating critical machine learning models in resource constrained regimes. In: International Conference on Medical Image Computing and Computer-Assisted Intervention, pp. 325–335. Springer, Cham (2023)
21. Shen, D., Wu, G., Suk, H.I.: Deep learning in medical image analysis. Annu. Rev. Biomed. Eng. **19**(1), 221–248 (2017)
22. Starmans, M., et al.: Reproducible radiomics through automated machine learning validated on twelve clinical applications. arXiv preprint arXiv:2108.08618 (2021)
23. Starmans, M.P., et al.: The WORC database: MRI and CT scans, segmentations, and clinical labels for 930 patients from six radiomics studies. medRxiv, pp. 2021–08 (2021)
24. Yang, L., Shami, A.: On hyperparameter optimization of machine learning algorithms: theory and practice. Neurocomputing **415**, 295–316 (2020)
25. Zhou, B., Khosla, A., Lapedriza, A., Oliva, A., Torralba, A.: Learning deep features for discriminative localization. In: Proceedings of the IEEE Conference on Computer Vision and Pattern Recognition, pp. 2921–2929 (2016)
26. Zhou, T., Ye, X., Lu, H., Zheng, X., Qiu, S., Liu, Y.: Dense convolutional network and its application in medical image analysis. Biomed. Res. Int. **2022**(1), 2384830 (2022)

Oral Presentations 3: Signals, Bias, and Structure in Medical Data

A Study in Scatter: Investigating Low-Contrast Image Contents Outside the X-Ray Collimation

Heiko Maier[1,2,3(✉)], Shahrooz Faghihroohi[1,2,3], Philipp Steininger[4], Amir Yousefi[5], Felix Wirth[6,7], Angelos Karlas[1,8,9], and Nassir Navab[1,3]

[1] Computer Aided Medical Procedures, Technical University of Munich, Munich, Germany

[2] Department of Cardiology, TUM University Hospital German Heart Center, Technical University of Munich, Munich, Germany
heiko.maier@tum.de

[3] Munich Center for Machine Learning (MCML), Munich, Germany

[4] medPhoton GmbH, Salzburg, Austria

[5] Department of Vascular Surgery, HELIOS Klinikum Munich West, Munich, Germany

[6] Department of Cardiovascular Surgery, TUM University Hospital German Heart Center, Technical University of Munich, Munich, Germany

[7] Institute INSURE, TUM University Hospital German Heart Center, Technical University of Munich, Munich, Germany

[8] Clinic and Polyclinic for Vascular and Endovascular Surgery, TUM University Hospital, Hospital rechts der Isar, Technical University of Munich, Munich, Germany

[9] DZHK, Partner Site Munich Heart Alliance, Munich, Germany

Abstract. Fluoroscopy is a widely used modality that provides vision to surgeons in minimally invasive surgery, but inherently raises concerns about radiation exposure. Collimation is a technique to reduce exposure by narrowing the radiation to a smaller area, with the trade-off of field-of-view limitations. However, the constraint the collimator shutters form for the x-ray beam is not absolute. Due to the non-ideal properties of the x-ray imaging and collimation process, small amounts of radiation are detectable outside the collimated area. This is a source of additional information, freely available as a byproduct of the imaging process, yet currently left unregarded. We explore whether this information can be used to provide additional knowledge about the surgical scene. In particular, we investigate whether it can be used to detect and visualize anatomical landmarks and surgical devices outside of the collimated area. We discuss the origins of this phenomenon, and perform experiments to evaluate its properties under different x-ray source parameters. Using anthropomorphic phantoms and a set of surgical guidewires, we investigate how well and under which conditions different landmarks and devices can be visualized with the proposed concept. We hope this work can open a path to provide additional information to interventional radiologists, while making use of every bit of radiation the patient is exposed to.

N. Akash et al. (Eds.): EMERGE 2025 Workshops, LNCS 16534, pp. 71–80, 2026.
https://doi.org/10.1007/978-3-032-24182-5_7

Keywords: X-Ray Imaging · Minimally Invasive Surgery · Interventional Radiology · Collimation

1 Introduction

In minimally invasive interventions, surgeons use fluoroscopy to visualize anatomical landmarks and surgical instruments inside the human body. As fluoroscopy is a live stream of X-ray images, it subjects both patient and clinical staff to radiation. A way to reduce the radiation dose is to narrow down the x-ray beam, so that it irradiates only the anatomical region of interest. This *collimation* is done by sliding metallic collimator shutters into the path between X-ray source and patient. The shutters form a window that constrains the emitted radiation to the area of interest, blocking rays that would irradiate the rest of the patient (Fig. 1a). Collimation decreases the radiation dose, with the trade-off of limiting the surgeon's field of view. In an idealized scenario, collimation would lead to a part of the X-ray detector being fully irradiated and the rest of the detector receiving no radiation at all, creating an image as in Fig. 1c. We explore subtle information contained in parts of the detector that are shielded by the collimator shutters - regions that would not receive any radiation based on the idealized scenario described above - and assess if such information can be used to alleviate the field of view limitation of collimation. We discuss the information's origins and explore its use to reconstruct shape and location of bones and surgical tools. Our contributions are to report the potential of this information for reconstructing bones and devices outside the collimated area; to investigate its characteristics in an imaging robot, and to introduce a method of histogram equalization and averaging to reconstruct bones and medical instruments in different scenarios.

To the best of our knowledge, we are the first to explore the potential this phenomenon could hold for reconstruction outside the collimated field of view.

2 Related Works

Common ways of dose reduction are automatic exposure/brightness control (AEC/ABC) to tune x-ray settings to each patient [14], pulsed fluoroscopy at low pulse rates [3,9,14] (or combined with electromagnetic tracking [7]), soft radiation filters [14], and last-image-hold (LIH) when the surgeon pauses fluoroscopy [9]. Also collimation [3,14] (e.g. AI-assisted for ROI selection [13]) reduces dose. During a procedure, the surgeon needs to see both anatomical landmarks, as well as the medical devices they currently manipulate inside the body. While static collimation to the overall anatomical region of interest can reduce radiation, stronger dose reduction is possible. Previous works proposed to collimate as narrowly as possible at each point in time, providing the surgeon with just enough information to perform the current step of the procedure. This is done by automatically finding the current region of interest (e.g. the location of a navigated surgical instrument) and dynamically changing the collimated image interval to

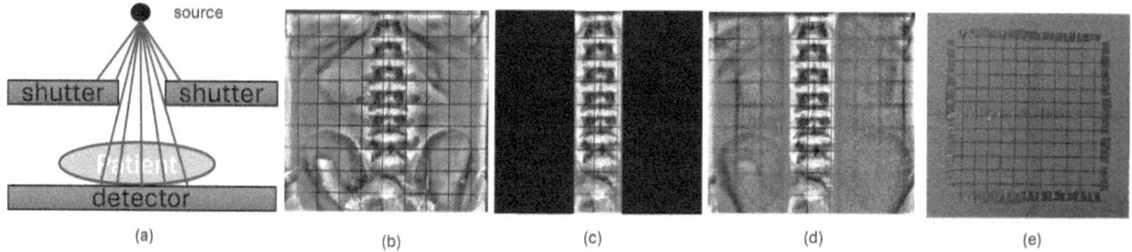

Fig. 1. (a) Collimated X-ray imaging; (b) uncollimated image of phantom #2 with guidewire grid on top; (c) idealized (artificial) collimated image, (d) a real collimated image with bone structures appearing in the regions outside the collimated area; (e) manufactured wire grid. (b), (c) and (d) postprocessed using histogram normalization.

encompass it [10]. While their approach reduced radiation, they recognized the risk that some information could be lost due to the reduced field of view from collimation. Therefore, they merged the constantly updated collimated image with uncollimated images taken at a lower framerate, opening up the collimator shutters once per second. This updates the peripheral image regions at a lower frequency than the central area - a compromise to retain full-field-of-view context while reducing radiation. A successful clinical use case of this method was shown as well [1]. Instead of temporally merging background and collimated frames, other works proposed to spatially modulate the emitted X-ray intensity by mounting a region-of-interest (ROI) attenuator, made of a copper plate with a central hole, in front of the X-ray source [2,11]. While the central beam is unimpeded, radiation to peripheral regions is reduced by around 80% [11] through the copper plate (different from collimator shutters that block almost all radiation from traversing). This provides the surgeon with a central image region benefiting from full X-ray exposure and sharp contrast and a peripheral image with lower contrast (and reduced radiation dose) to retain full-field of view.

Both temporal and spatial approaches aim at dose reduction while preserving full field of view. Compared to these works, we are interested in whether we can reconstruct information from regions outside the collimated area without having to un- and recollimate (as in [10]) and without modifying the device as in [11], using information naturally emerging from the image formation process. We are specifically interested in features in the regions of collimated images that correspond to parts of the detector shielded by the collimator shutters. A collimated X-ray image consists of two parts: the central, *collimated region* between the shutters and the *shielded region* outside the collimated area. The collimated region stems from the parts of the detector that directly receive radiation from the source, geometrically determined by a theoretical point source irradiating the X-rays and the window formed by the collimator shutters. Under the idealized assumptions of a) a point radiation source, b) collimator shutters entirely blocking incoming radiation, and c) no scattering events, these are the only parts of the detector receiving radiation from the source, creating an image as in Fig. 1c. The collimator shutters block direct radiation from reaching the shielded regions.

However, the image formation process (see e.g. [4]) is non-ideal. The X-ray source is not a point source; it has a finite focal spot distribution, creating additional off-focal spot radiation [5]. Also, scattering events occur inside the X-ray tube, the collimator, and the patient. These effects form a distribution of sources. Most interestingly, this leads to image information outside the collimated regions. A reconstruction of such information in the shielded regions using local histogram equalization [12] is visualized in Fig. 1d. Strongly attenuating structures, such as bones, are visible in regions outside of the collimated area.

3 Materials and Methods

We experimentally confirmed and evaluated this with Loop-X, a mobile imaging robot. We collected native, raw detector images (1440×1440). Collimator shutters of Loop-X are proven radio-intransparent (>99.9% absorption [8]), so our results are not due to X-rays penetrating the collimator. We were interested in visibility of bones or medical devices in the shielded regions. To investigate device visibility across different image parts all at once, we used Amplatz Extra Stiff Guidewires (diameter 0.89 mm, Cook Medical), routinely used endovascular surgical instruments. We cut the wires and manufactured a 30×30 cm grid on cardboard, with 2.5 cm spacing (Fig. 1e). As shielded regions only receive radiation with an intensity far smaller than the main beam's, information in those regions is noisy and image features have poor contrast. We visualize this information using local histogram equalization (CLAHE [12], radius 71, $\alpha = \beta = 0.0$).

4 Experiments

We performed 3 sets of experiments to investigate different influencing factors.

Open Beam Properties. We evaluated the raw image intensity distributions on the detector when the beam is collimated, but no object is placed between detector and source; to isolate the imaging system's influence on information in the shielded regions from other sources like phantom scatter. We assessed the influence of several parameters on this distribution in the shielded regions. Geometric parameters were size, position and aspect ratio of the collimation box. Exposure parameters were tube current, voltage and focal spot size (Loop-X offers 0.3 mm and 0.6 mm). Tube current was 0.5 mA or 1.0 mA; voltage 80 or 120 kV. This low current setting avoids overexposure while no object attenuates the beam. For each exposure setting, we tested a set of box sizes, either collimated to the center of the detector, or to the point opposite the focal spot of the source (where the central line of the X-ray beam hits the detector). For some settings we sampled more box positions and varied box anisotropy. We always took an uncollimated reference image. For each image, we recorded 11 frames of 84 ms.

Wire Grid. To test how the results of the first experiment translate to visibility of medical devices, we took collimated images with a wire grid in the X-ray beam.

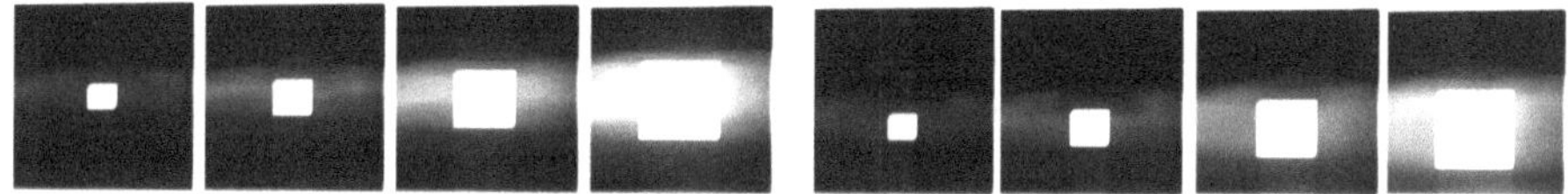

Fig. 2. Irradiation patterns of collimation boxes, at 120 kV, 0.5 mA with a large focal spot. Left cluster is centered to detector center, right is opposite to focal spot. Each pixel represents the percentage of radiation the respective detector cell recorded compared to an uncollimated image. Images are cropped to [0.0, 0.05] for visibility (white detector regions still recorded $\geq$ 5% of the uncollimated radiation intensity despite being behind collimator shutters). Central white squares are the collimated area, outside regions indicate radiation in shielded areas.

Anthropomorphic Phantoms. We used two anthropomorphic X-ray torso phantoms (The Phantom Laboratory & Kyoto Kagaku) for our final experiment. Phantom #1 contains a human skeleton cast into a material with the same effective atomic number as human soft tissue. Phantom #2 consists of resins (radiological absorption and HU number comparable to the human body). We recorded collimated images with the wire grid on top of the phantoms, in different exposure and geometric parameterizations. Default source parameters were 120 kV, 4.0 mA, anterior-posterior (AP) orientation, large focal spot.

5 Results and Discussion

As information in shielded regions is noisy, we present results obtained by averaging 11 frames (slightly less than 1 s of Fluoroscopy), unless stated otherwise.

Open Beam Properties. We confirmed residual radiation in the shielded regions. To understand its magnitude, we divided each collimated image by an uncollimated reference image. Thereby, we obtained for each pixel the percentage of intensity recorded during collimation compared to the intensity without collimation. For two sets of square collimation boxes, the results are shown in Fig. 2. As expected due to the orientation of the rotating anode [5], we found that radiation in the shielded regions is much more prevalent in the horizontal axis. Only little residual radiation could be found in the vertical direction. With increasing box size, the irradiated area both grows wider and the intensity inside of it increases. For two different box positions (detector center and opposite focal spot), this pattern was comparable, though the exact shape shows some dependency on position. We present results from different x-ray source parameters in Fig. 3a. Lower tube voltage (80 kV) showed increased radiation in the shielded areas compared to 120 kV across the whole detector. Focal spot size impacted the irradiation pattern locally, but did not overall increase or decrease the amount of radiation in the shielded regions. Results for anisotropic boxes spanning the whole detector width or height are shown in Fig. 3b. Column-wise collimation showed prevalence of irradiation in the upper half of the detector, and that radiation extended further toward the left than to the right when collimating

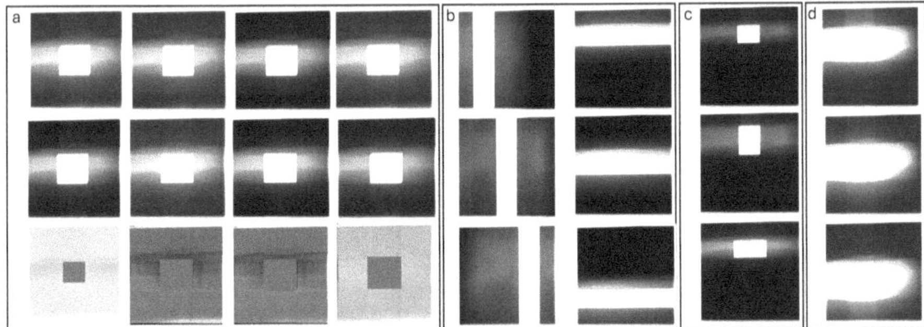

Fig. 3. (a) Comparison of tube settings. In each column, the first and second image are two different settings and the third is the difference between them. For visibility, images are cropped to a range of [0.0, 0.05] and difference images to [−0.01, 0.01]. In difference images, the center is set to 0.0 to provide a reference of regions with increased intensity (brighter than center) or decreased (darker). From left to right: 80 kV vs 120 kV tube voltage at (0.5 mA-large FS); Large vs small focal spot at (80 kV–0.5 mA), Large vs small focal spot at (120 kV–0.5 mA), 0.5 mA vs 1.0 mA at (80 kV-large FS. (b) Images obtained with different column and row collimations (c) different aspect ratios (d) influence of box size on vertical collimation beam (images cropped to [0.0, 0.02].

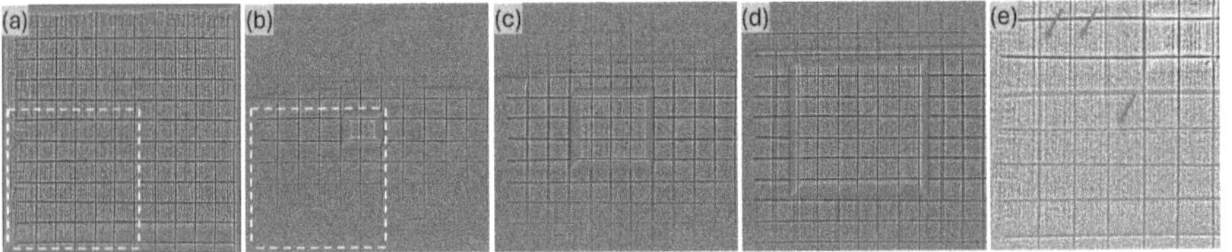

Fig. 4. Wire Grid with different collimation sizes, (a) uncollimated (b) 5 cm (c) 12.5 cm (d) 22.5 cm. (e) zoomed-in overlay of part (yellow outline) of (a) and (b). CLAHE 11×11 (Color figure online).

off-center. Row-wise collimation confirmed that vertically, not much radiation is found. Results for smaller anisotropic boxes are in Fig. 3c. Extending boxes vertically lead to a larger shielded area being affected. Horizontal extension increased the intensity in the affected areas. Vertical box position also slightly influenceed the vertical irradiation pattern, extending away from the center (Fig. 3d).

Wire Grid. The grid could successfully be visualized in the shielded regions, with characteristics similar to the open beam experiments, most notably the horizontal prevalence. Interestingly, while larger collimated boxes did increase the irradiated area as expected, they also increasingly blurred the wires (Fig. 4). Additionally, a geometric deformation was observed: the reconstructed wires were shifted compared to their uncollimated position (see overlay in Fig. 4e). We attribute this to the fact that the information in shielded regions comes from off-focal and scattered radiation. Deformation grew with distance from center. *Anthropomorphic Phantom* In the anthropomorphic phantoms, we investigated the interplay of tissue properties and visibility of bones and devices. In Phantom #1, in AP recording, we could successfully visualize both wires and certain bones in the shielded regions (Fig. 5a, Images 1,2,3). Visibility depended on total attenuation in the path through the body, with e.g. ribs being easier to recover in front of lungs (Fig. 5a, region R1 in red) than in front of abdominal tissue (Fig. 5a, region R2). Similarly, wires were clearly visible in front of lungs and ribs, yet visibility decreased in front of soft tissue. Wires overlapping with the spine were barely noticeable (Fig. 5a, img. 4 & 5, R3). The finding from open beam experiments that radiation extends more toward the left than to the right for off-center collimation was also seen here (Fig 5a, img. 4 vs 5). A higher number of averaged frames visualized bones and wires more finely (Fig. 5a, img. 2 & 3), also when they suffer from reduced visibility due to attenuating tissue or bones. Smaller collimation boxes showed the same horizontal preference as in the open beam experiments, combined with the finding from the wire grid experiments that larger boxes blurred wires more than small ones (Fig. 5a, Image 6).

In phantom #2, we found that higher tube voltage lead to sharper, more distinguishable image features for ribs, hips (Fig. 5b, tube voltage section, red arrows) and wires. Lowering tube current from 4 mA to 2 mA reduced clarity (Fig. 5b, tube current section). To evaluate wire sharpness and contrast, we calculated the wires' full width at half maximum (FWHM) and contrast-to-noise ratio (CNR). FWHM was computed on a gaussian ($\sigma = 1.0$) and median filtered (kernel 7) average of 100 rows (center and boundaries shown as yellow lines in Fig. 5b). CNR was calculated from an unfiltered patch consisting of the same 100 rows. The CNR signal level was calculated as mean of the region ±0.5*FWHM around the center (peak) of the wire. CNR noise level and standard deviation were estimated from regions ±2.5–4.0*FWHM left and right of the center. Mean wire FWHM and CNR are stated above the images in Fig. 5b. Comparing AP orientation of source and detector with PA orientation (Fig. 5b, orientation section), we found the grid to be sharper in PA. This likely results from the grid being closer to the detector in PA setting, leading to lower magnification and higher image clarity. Geometric deformation was again observed, mostly horizontal (Fig. 5c).

In some procedures, guidewires move in the abdominal aorta above the spine. Thus, we explored if we could visualize wires even in front of the spine. To align the horizontal irradiation pattern with the spine, we rotated the phantom by 90°. We chose a small collimation box, as would be the case if focusing on the tip of a guidewire, which as we know from above results also produces sharper features than a larger collimation box. We could visualize the wire in multiple scenarios. In AP orentation, for 120 kV, the wire could be visualized, but visualization was poor at 90 kV (Fig. 5d, section recording in AP). In PA, we could visualize the wire at 90 kV, with clarity increasing for more averaged frames (Fig. 5d, section recording in PA). For reference, a study in endovascular abdominal interventions reported 3.1 mA and 81 kV as low-dose protocol [6], so our parameters of 2.0 to 4.0 mA and 80 to 120 kV are in a reasonable range for minimally invasive surgery.

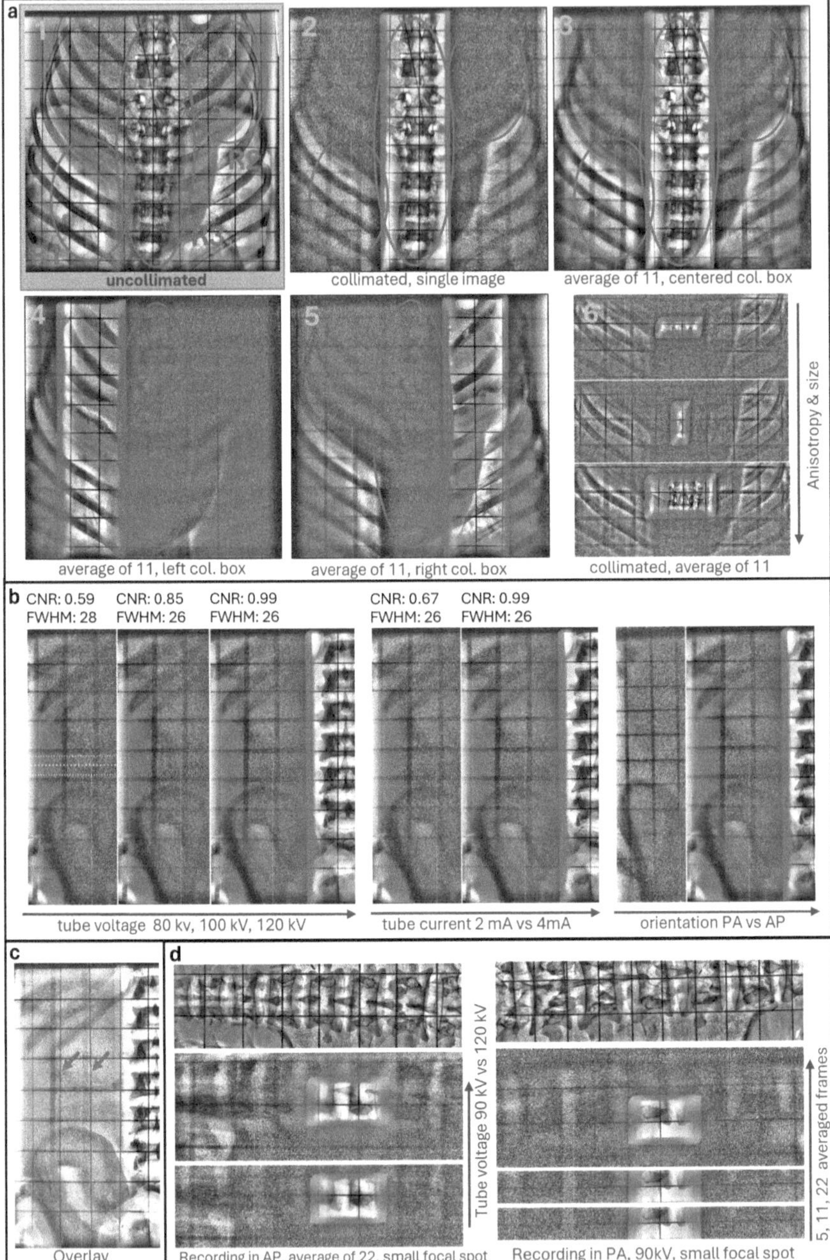

Fig. 5. Various phantom+grid images, CLAHE filtered (a) phantom #1 (head-down), analysing averaging, box position and size, (b) tube voltage, current and orientation in abdominal area of phantom #2 (uncollimated image in Fig. 1b) (c) overlay showing geometric deformation (d) cropped view of spine of phantom #2; phantom rotated to align with dominant axis of radiation, comparing orientation, averaging and voltage.

6 Conclusion

We introduced and explored the use of information contained in shielded regions of collimated images in order to reconstruct bones and surgical devices outside of the collimated area. This concept is of interest because in clinical settings, radiation protection and procedural safety are both crucial. We envision our approach integrated into a system that tracks and collimates to the tip of the device the surgeon currently manipulates, which is the most important part of the device they need to see. Narrow collimation to the tip would reduce patient dose, yet there are important warning signs the surgeon might miss - e.g. if outside the collimated area the device loops or kinks along the shaft. Also, if during advancement and tracking of a stent graft system over a wire, the end of the wire is unintentionally advanced (e.g. into the heart during TEVAR), the surgeon must know. Or if an already placed therapeutic device (e.g. stent graft) dislodges while he manipulates another device. Finally, instead of relying only on a small collimation window, reconstruction of bones could help to ensure that registration with a static model (2D contrast run or 3D CTA) stays accurate in case of patient motion, e.g. in PAD intervention with local anesthesia. Providing awareness about the surgical scene, while reducing radiation by narrow collimation, is thus a clinical setting that would benefit from our approach.

The results of our initial investigation indicate that this concept has potential to alleviate some of the field-of-view limitations of collimated imaging while inducing no additional radiation to the patient. Yet, it is also clear that each potential application has to be carefully chosen, due to spatial characteristics like the horizontal prevalence or interaction of devices with highly attenuating structures like the spine. The averaging needs to use previously acquired frames, as new exposures would increase dose. Thus, temporal influences of averaging frames during patient or instrument motion need to be considered. We hope this work inspires researchers and device manufacturers to explore this concept.

Acknowledgments. Heiko Maier is supported by TUM International Graduate School of Science and Engineering (IGSSE). We thank BrainLab AG for their partial support.

Disclosure of Interests. Philipp Steininger is co-owner of medPhoton GmbH. Other authors have no competing interests.

References

1. Bang, J.Y., Hough, M., Hawes, R.H., Varadarajulu, S.: Use of artificial intelligence to reduce radiation exposure at fluoroscopy-guided endoscopic procedures. Am. J. Gastroenterol. **115**(4), 555–561 (2020). https://doi.org/10.14309/ajg.0000000000000565
2. Borota, L., Patz, A.: Spot region of interest imaging: a novel functionality aimed at X-ray dose reduction in neurointerventional procedures. Radiat. Prot. Dosimetry. **188**(3), 322–331 (2020). https://doi.org/10.1093/rpd/ncz290

3. Bousis, C., Kosovitsas, T., Karanikis, P., Kotsia, A., Tzima, E., Pappa, E.: Dose-area product reduction through a practice implementing low frame rate fluoroscopy and increased collimation during single-vessel percutaneous coronary interventions. Radiat. Prot. Environ. **47**(2) (2024). https://doi.org/10.4103/rpe.rpe_13_24
4. Haidekker, M.A.: Medical Imaging Technology. Springer (2013). https://doi.org/10.1007/978-1-4614-7073-1
5. van der Heyden, B., et al.: Modelling of the focal spot intensity distribution and the off-focal spot radiation in kilovoltage X-ray tubes for imaging. Phys. Med. Biol. **65**(2), 025002 (2020). https://doi.org/10.1088/1361-6560/ab6178
6. Kalef-Ezra, J.A., Karavasilis, S., Ziogas, D., Dristiliaris, D., Michalis, L.K., Matsagas, M.: Radiation burden of patients undergoing endovascular abdominal aortic aneurysm repair. J. Vasc. Surg. **49**(2), 283–287 (2009). https://doi.org/10.1016/j.jvs.2008.09.003
7. Krumb, H.J., Dorweiler, B., Mukhopadhyay, A.: Hex: a safe research framework for hybrid EMT X-ray navigation. Int. J. Comput. Assist. Radiol. Surg. **18**(7), 1175–1183 (2023). https://doi.org/10.1007/s11548-023-02917-y
8. medPhoton GmbH: User Manual ImagingRing m/Loop-X (2025). https://www.medphoton.at/user-manuals/, version 30.1. Accessed 29 July 2025
9. Mitchell, E.L., Furey, P.: Prevention of radiation injury from medical imaging. J. Vasc. Surg. **53**(1, Suppl.), 22S–27S (2011). https://doi.org/10.1016/j.jvs.2010.05.139
10. Nir, G., et al.: Automatic detection and tracking of the region of interest during fluoroscopy-guided procedures for radiation exposure reduction. In: Medical Imaging 2021: Image-Guided Procedures, Robotic Interventions, and Modeling. Society of Photo-Optical Instrumentation Engineers (SPIE) Conference Series, vol. 11598, p. 1159828 (2021). https://doi.org/10.1117/12.2580729
11. Orji, M.P., Williams, K., Nagesh, S.S., Rudin, S., Bednarek, D.R.: Fluoroscopic procedure-room scatter-dose reduction using a region-of-interest (ROI) attenuator. In: Medical Imaging 2024: Physics of Medical Imaging, vol. 12925, pp. 749–758. SPIE (2024). https://doi.org/10.1117/12.3006856
12. Pizer, S.M., et al.: Adaptive histogram equalization and its variations. Comput. Vis. Graph. Image Process. **39**(3), 355–368 (1987). https://doi.org/10.1016/S0734-189X(87)80186-X
13. Ravi, A., et al.: Optimizing neurointerventional procedures: an algorithm for embolization coil detection and automated collimation to enable dose reduction. J. Med. Imaging **11**(4), 044003 (2024). https://doi.org/10.1117/1.JMI.11.4.044003
14. Walters, T.E., Kistler, P.M., Morton, J.B., Sparks, P.B., Halloran, K., Kalman, J.M.: Impact of collimation on radiation exposure during interventional electrophysiology. EP Europace **14**(11), 1670–1673 (2012). https://doi.org/10.1093/europace/eus095

ESCAViT: Symmetry-Aware EEG Classification

Se Hwan Lim[1,2] and Hyun Gyu Lee[3,4](✉)

[1] Department of Electronic Engineering, Inha University, Incheon, Republic of Korea
tpghks726@inha.edu

[2] Department of Artificial Intelligence Semiconductor Engineering, Inha University, Incheon, Republic of Korea

[3] Department of Electrical and Computer Engineering, Inha University, Incheon, Republic of Korea
hglee@inha.ac.kr

[4] College of Medicine, Inha University, Incheon, Republic of Korea

Abstract. Accurate classification of Ictal-Interictal-Injury Continuum (IIIC) patterns is essential for neurological assessment in intensive care units, yet remains challenging due to limitations in capturing inter-lead correlations and addressing class imbalance. To tackle this, we propose ESCAViT, a multi-stream Transformer-based EEG classification framework. ESCAViT leverages the Video Vision Transformer with specialized feature extraction mechanisms to model spatiotemporal EEG patterns, while applying domain-adaptive learning to enhance data diversity and mitigate heterogeneous Other class (HOC) effects. Experimental results on the IIIC dataset show that ESCAViT outperforms state-improvement in mean accuracy per class (mACC) and **22.6%** in F1-score. Our method significantly enhances LRDA classification **by over 20%**, thereby addressing classification bias. ESCAViT demonstrates consistent performance across different IIIC patterns and imbalanced distributions, confirming its effectiveness in EEG classification. The code is available at https://github.com/limshmai/ESCAViT.git.

Keywords: IIIC Pattern Classification · EEG Transformer · Inter-Lead Contrastive Learning · Class Imbalance Mitigation

1 Introduction

Electroencephalogram (EEG) monitoring plays a vital role in detecting and managing neurological injuries in intensive care units (ICUs) [1]. Among various EEG patterns, IIIC patterns are frequently observed in critically ill patients. These patterns, which include Seizure, Lateralized Periodic Discharges (LPD), Generalized Periodic Discharges (GPD), Lateralized Rhythmic Delta Activity (LRDA), and Generalized Rhythmic Delta Activity (GRDA), provide crucial diagnostic insights into subclinical seizures and seizure-like electrical events, aiding early neurological injury detection [2].

N. Akash et al. (Eds.): EMERGE 2025 Workshops, LNCS 16534, pp. 81–90, 2026.
https://doi.org/10.1007/978-3-032-24182-5_8

However, IIIC pattern classification remains challenging due to two key factors:

1. Inter-lead relationships & spatial dependencies–In IIIC classification, Lateralized patterns are confined to one hemisphere, while Generalized patterns manifest symmetrically across both hemispheres. This hemispheric symmetry is crucial for distinguishing seizures from non-ictal activity, yet existing methods fail to effectively model these inter-lead correlations [3,4].
2. Data ambiguity & class imbalance–Expert disagreement and severe class imbalance (Other: 7,205 vs. LRDA: 936) introduce significant classification bias [5,6].

To address these challenges, we propose ESCAViT, a multi-stream Transformer-based EEG classification framework that explicitly models EEG lead symmetry and enhances feature robustness through domain-adaptive learning. Unlike conventional Video Vision Transformer (ViViT) architecture [7], which struggles with local representation, ESCAViT introduces the following key contributions:

1. **Lead-Aware Feature Extraction:** Pairwise Attention and Lead Attention are incorporated to explicitly capture inter-lead dependencies, improving spatial-temporal EEG representation.
2. **Domain-Specific Learning Strategies:** To mitigate class imbalance and HOC issues and enhance feature generalization, we design a unified framework that integrates Adaptive EEG Spectrogram Mixup (AES-Mix) and Lead Interrelation-Guided Contrastive Learning (LIGCL).
3. **Multi-Pathway Feature Integration:** Overlapping Convolutional Projection and Multi-Stream Architecture enable fine-grained seizure pattern detection while preserving global EEG structure.

Through these innovations, ESCAViT significantly enhances IIIC pattern classification, particularly in capturing symmetrical relationships between left and right hemisphere leads, outperforming existing methods.

2 Related Work

EEG classification presents unique challenges due to its high-dimensional, noisy, and ambiguous nature, making traditional spectrum analysis and wavelet-based methods suboptimal [8]. Recent deep learning approaches have demonstrated superior performance across various EEG-related tasks, including seizure detection and neurodegenerative disease diagnosis [9].

Hybrid GNN-CNN Models.. Hybrid GNN-CNN models [3] and spatial multi-scale attention mechanisms [10] have been introduced to address these limitations. However, these methods still face challenges in modeling dynamic feature interactions due to the structural rigidity of GNN-based graph representations.

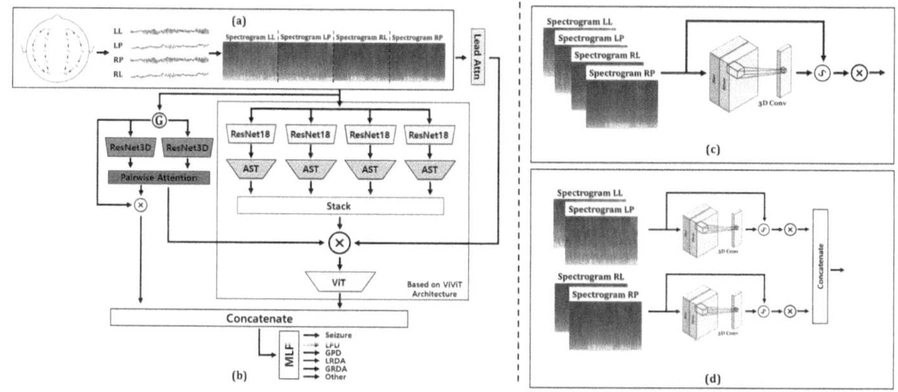

Fig. 1. Architecture of ESCAViT. (a) EEG preprocessing: 20 raw leads compressed into four key leads (LL, LP, RL, RP) and converted to Mel-Spectrograms. (b) ESCAViT structure: integration of ViViT-based inter-channel modeling and hemisphere-specific 3D ResNet pathways. (c) Lead-Attention and (d) Pairwise Attention mechanisms for modeling inter-lead relationships and enhancing spatial-spectral feature extraction.

Transformer-Based EEG Analysis. Transformers leverage self-attention mechanisms for long-range feature extraction [4], yet lack explicit spatial priors, limiting their ability to model local EEG variations and inter-lead correlations. ViT-based architectures [11] show promise in EEG classification but struggle to capture fine-grained seizure morphology changes.

Motivation for ESCAViT. Existing EEG models fail to comprehensively address lead symmetry, class imbalance, and data ambiguity. To resolve these issues, we propose ESCAViT, which integrates ViViT-based multi-stream feature learning with domain-specific techniques for effective IIIC pattern classification.

3 Methodology

3.1 Overview

The preprocessing pipeline of ESCAViT comprises two stages, as illustrated in Fig. 1(a). Initially, the Banana Montage technique [12] reduces the original 20 EEG leads to four key leads (LL, LP, RL, RP), thereby reducing computational complexity while preserving spatial relationships. Subsequently, each lead is transformed into a Mel-Spectrogram [13] with a temporal axis of 256 s to facilitate time-frequency analysis. In the lead notation, the first letter denotes the Left/Right hemisphere, while the second letter indicates the Lateral/Parasagittal position.

As shown in Fig. 1(b) and (c), (d), ESCAViT integrates ViViT-based inter-channel modeling with hemisphere-specific spatiotemporal feature extraction to overcome the limitations of conventional ViViT models. The architecture consists of a ViViT-based pathway for global feature extraction and two 3D ResNet pathways that independently learn spatiotemporal EEG representations from each cerebral hemisphere. Convolutional Projection and Lead Attention mechanisms are incorporated to explicitly capture inter-lead dependencies. Additionally, ESCAViT applies a unified framework that integrates AES-Mix for data augmentation and LIGCL for contrastive learning to improve class separability and robustness against data ambiguity.

3.2 Feature Extraction with Lead Attention

Seizure EEG signals are characterized by the sudden appearance of distinct spectral patterns at specific time points. To effectively capture these temporal and spectral fluctuations, we propose a Lead Attention mechanism based on spatial attention [14]. Unlike CBAM, which employs 2D spatial pooling, Lead Attention explicitly models inter-lead dependencies and EEG-specific time-frequency variations while preserving temporal information through 3D convolutions.

Lead Attention dynamically learns the importance of four leads at each time frame. By extracting mean and maximum values from the time-frequency representations of each lead and generating attention weights through 3D convolutions, the mechanism can selectively focus on specific leads exhibiting seizure activity. Pairwise Attention groups left hemisphere leads (LL, LP) and right hemisphere leads (RL, RP) to explicitly model inter-hemispheric symmetry.

For lead-wise feature extraction, the AST architecture employs DeiT-Base (12 layers, 768 dimensions, 12 attention heads) applied to each lead, dividing mel-spectrograms into 16×16 patches. Unlike standard AST models, ESCAViT incorporates Overlapping Convolutional Projection to overcome the limitations of ViT-based models in capturing fine-grained seizure morphology [15,16]. As illustrated in Fig. 1(d), Lead Attention extracts mean and maximum values along the frequency and time axes and generates attention weights through a 3D convolutional network. These weights refine the AST-based representations to enhance localized seizure pattern detection.

3.3 Feature Integration

Extracted features from each lead are integrated using a Global Feature Transformer (Fig. 1(b)), which is a ViT-Base model pretrained on ImageNet. The Global Feature Transformer integrates four leads as 2×1 patches and employs learnable absolute position embeddings at all stages. This integration leverages Convolutional Projection [16] for enhanced local feature encoding and overlapping patch embeddings to maintain critical long-range dependencies.

Pairwise Attention (Fig. 1(c)) models hemispheric relationships by distinguishing left-right asymmetries, thereby improving seizure pattern detection. Through these mechanisms, ESCAViT effectively integrates spatial and spectral EEG features, outperforming traditional methods in capturing inter-lead dependencies.

Table 1. Comparison of EEG models on IIIC classification performance. 1D models are trained on raw EEG data, while 2D models use EEG spectrograms as input features.

Input	Model Type	Method	ACC	F1	KLD	TPS	mACC
1D	Graph	1D GNN-CNN [19]	0.394	0.246	0.830	0.192	0.248
	Transformer	EEG Conformer [20]	0.351	0.298	0.869	0.337	0.341
	1D-based	SPaRCNet [21]	0.636	0.546	0.698	0.447	0.511
2D	Transformer	AST(Tiny) [15]	0.503	0.421	0.766	0.378	0.411
		w/ DRT	0.554	0.462	0.741	0.453	0.457
	Domain-Adaptive Learning	DANN [22]	0.495	0.280	0.816	0.163	0.284
		w/ DRT	0.659	0.556	0.714	0.539	0.552
3D	3D CNN	ResNet3D [23]	0.670	0.600	0.670	0.576	0.592
		w/ DRT	0.744	0.684	0.623	0.692	0.685
	Ours	ESCAViT(base)	0.719	0.662	0.628	0.663	0.653
		ESCAViT(w/ DRT)	**0.758**	**0.714**	**0.605**	**0.700**	**0.704**

3.4 Domain Robust Technique

ESCAViT integrates two domain-adaptive learning strategies, AES-Mix and LIGCL, to address data ambiguity, HOC issues, and class imbalance in EEG classification. Each technique targets specific challenges through complementary mechanisms.

AES-Mix addresses class imbalance by selectively augmenting minority classes (LPD, GRDA, LRDA) to resolve feature learning failures in underrepresented patterns [17]. Since RDA exhibit diagnostic features in 1–4 Hz band, mixing is restricted to this range to preserve critical characteristics [18].

LIGCL targets data ambiguity from low inter-rater agreement through adaptive contrastive learning. It uses mixup ratio λ as weights–higher for original-like samples to maintain boundaries, lower for mixed samples to control ambiguity.

Their synergistic integration overcomes individual limitations: AES-Mix alone dilutes majority class features while LIGCL alone over-sharpens minority class boundaries. Combined, they enable robust performance on imbalanced and ambiguous IIIC patterns.

4 Experimental Results

4.1 Dataset and Experimental Setup

We used the publicly available harmful brain activity in electroencephalography (EEG) dataset (https://www.kaggle.com/competitions/hms-harmful-brain-activity-classification, [24]). The dataset consists of 17,089 EEG segments from 2,711 patients, annotated by 20 neurophysiology experts into five IIIC-related patterns (Seizure, LPD, GPD, LRDA, GRDA) and an Other category.

The dataset exhibits severe class imbalance, with the Other class comprising 42% while LRDA accounts for only 5%. Expert agreement varies significantly across patterns, with LRDA and GPD showing the lowest consensus (0.73 and

0.80, respectively), indicating high inter-observer variability. These imbalances and ambiguities highlight the necessity for domain-adaptive learning strategies.

For the experimental setup, we divided the 17,089 samples into training, validation, and testing sets using stratified splitting in an 8:1:1 ratio. All models were trained on one NVIDIA GeForce RTX A6000 48GB GPU using the AdamW optimizer with a learning rate of 1e-4, weight decay of 1e-3, batch size of 8, and 50 epochs.

4.2 Baseline Models and Evaluation Metrics

ESCAViT was evaluated against five types of state-of-the-art EEG classification models. These include 1D-based approaches (SPaRCNet [21]), graph-based models (GNN-CNN [19]), Transformer-based architectures (EEG Conformer [20], AST [15]), domain-adaptive learning (DANN [22]), and 3D CNN (ResNet3D [23]).

$$\mathrm{TPS} = \frac{\sum_i \mathbb{1}(\mathrm{pred}_i = \mathrm{true}_i) \cdot \mathbb{1}(\mathrm{class}_i \neq \mathrm{other})}{\sum_i \mathbb{1}(\mathrm{class}_i \neq \mathrm{other})} \tag{1}$$

To assess model performance, we used multiple metrics including Accuracy (ACC), macro-averaged F1-score, Mean Accuracy per Class (mACC), Target Pattern Sensitivity (TPS), and KL Divergence (KLD). The mACC [25] measures per-class accuracy to mitigate majority-class bias effects. TPS (Eq. 1) evaluates classification accuracy excluding the majority Other class, focusing on IIIC-related patterns. These two metrics served as primary indicators for evaluating classification performance under class imbalance.

4.3 Performance Evaluation and Comparative Analysis

As shown in Table 1, conventional 1D and 2D models struggle with IIIC pattern classification due to their limited ability to capture lead symmetry and seizure-specific patterns. Even SpaRCNet, a model specialized for IIIC, shows prediction bias with mACC and TPS below 51%. ResNet3D improves performance by leveraging spatial correlations but remains suboptimal due to its limitations in long-range feature extraction. In contrast, ESCAViT effectively captures inter-lead features through Pairwise Attention and ViViT-based architecture while extracting local features of seizure patterns via AST transfer learning, Lead Attention, and Convolutional Projection. This results in average performance improvements of 25.6% in F1, 30% in TPS, and 25.2% in mACC, demonstrating its ability to effectively capture seizure patterns while learning inter-lead correlations.

DRT further improves ESCAViT, achieving over 70% in mACC and TPS, confirming its effectiveness in mitigating prediction bias. Notably, DRT also enhances other spectrogram-based models, with DANN achieving a 16% accuracy increase. This demonstrates DRT's robustness in handling data ambiguity and class imbalance.

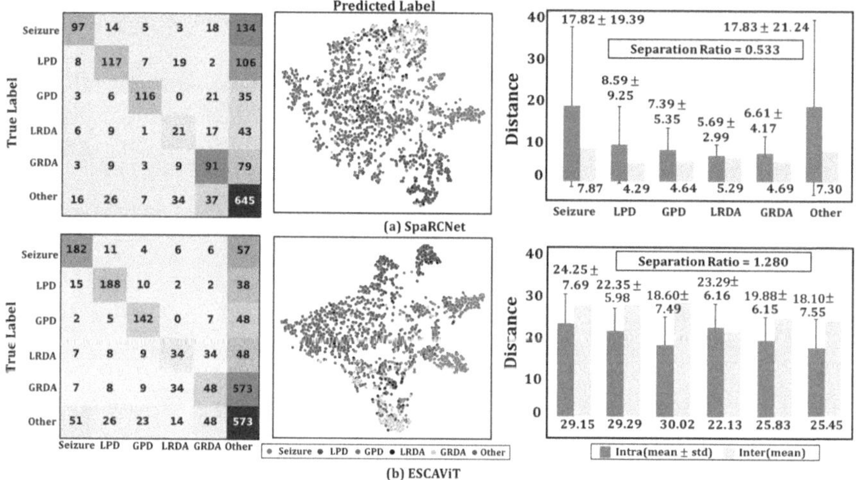

Fig. 2. Quantitative and qualitative comparison of models. (a) SpaRCNet from Table 1, (b) ESCAViT Base. Each model shows confusion matrix, t-SNE projection, and cluster-separation bar plot. Bar plots report mean intra-class distance (dark bars, ± 1 SD), mean inter-class distance (light bars), and separation ratio (inter/intra distance). Separation Ratio > 1 indicates well-separated clusters.

4.4 Visualization of Model Behavior

We analyzed model behavior using confusion matrices, T-SNE visualizations, and cluster-separation bar plots (Fig. 2). Compared to SpaRCNet, ESCAViT significantly reduced misclassifications into the Other class (397 → 187) and achieved 31.4% improvement in seizure classification through Lead Attention and Convolutional Projection. Pairwise Attention enhanced inter-lead symmetry modeling, reducing LRDA-GRDA misclassification errors from 26 to 19.

The superior cluster separation performance of ESCAViT was confirmed through T-SNE visualizations and bar plots. SpaRCNet exhibited high variance in intra-class cohesion (intra metric), while ESCAViT achieved smaller Intra-Distance than Inter-Distance for all classes except LRDA, demonstrating high intra-class cohesion. ESCAViT achieved a separation ratio 0.747 points higher than SpaRCNet.

Occlusion sensitivity analysis [26] (Fig. 3) confirmed ESCAViT's ability to capture hemispheric relationships. Unlike ResNet3D, which fails to consider left-right correlations, ESCAViT effectively highlights symmetrical EEG features, improving classification of ambiguous patterns.

4.5 Ablation Study

To confirm that the interaction between AES-Mix and LIGCL is essential in the proposed DRT, we conducted experiments by individually applying each

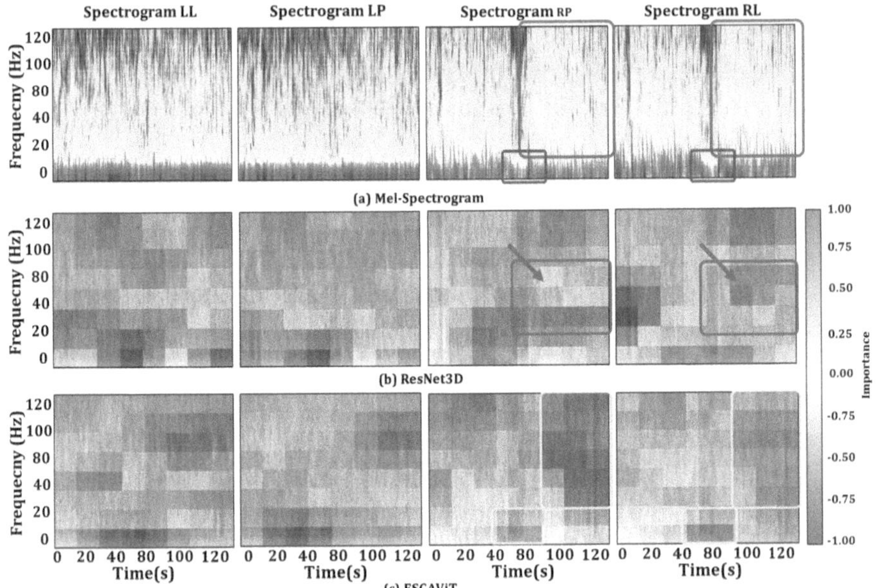

Fig. 3. Occlusion sensitivity analysis (patch size: 32×32, stride: 16×16). (a) Mel-Spectrogram visualization of an LRDA sample. Black boxes indicate regions where frequency and amplitude differences are observed between left and right channels. Right and left signals show similar patterns within each hemisphere. (b) ResNet3D and (c) ESCAViT feature importance heatmaps. Red boxes show ResNet3D assigning different importance values to the same time-frequency regions within right signals. Green boxes highlight ESCAViT assigning consistent importance, effectively capturing inter-lead symmetry. (Color figure online)

Table 2. Performance comparison of individual and combined application of AES-Mix and LIGCL in the proposed DRT. DRT represents the combined use of both techniques, while w/o AES-Mix indicates LIGCL only and w/o LIGCL indicates AES-Mix only. OthACC represents the accuracy of the Other class, which is the majority class.

Method	ACC	F1	KLD	TPS	mACC	OthACC
DRT	**0.758**	**0.714**	**0.605**	**0.700**	**0.704**	**0.795**
w/o AES-Mix	0.707	0.654	0.639	0.683	0.666	0.764
w/o LIGCL	0.723	0.663	0.628	0.692	0.652	0.741

technique to ESCAViT (base). As shown in Table 2, individual application of each technique resulted in performance degradation. When only AES-Mix was applied, insufficient representation of the Other class led to approximately a 5.4% decrease in majority class accuracy. Conversely, applying only LIGCL caused excessive boundary sharpening, resulting in a 5.2% decline in mACC score. This demonstrates that only the combined application of both techniques in DRT can effectively address class imbalance and enhance model performance.

5 Conclusions

In this paper, we propose ESCAViT, a ViViT-based model for IIIC pattern classification. To enhance inter-lead correlation learning, we introduce AST Transfer Learning, Convolutional Projection, and Lead Attention mechanisms, along with a DRT combining AES-Mix and LIGCL to address data ambiguity and class imbalance. Experimental results demonstrate that the proposed model achieves superior performance in classification and seizure pattern recognition compared to existing approaches. DRT effectively mitigates class imbalance and strengthens model generalization across diverse EEG patterns. ESCAViT shows how domain-adaptive modeling of biosignals can enhance the reliability of clinical decision support tools and contribute to developing generalizable AI systems suitable for real-world clinical deployment. For future work, we plan to validate the model's robustness on large-scale clinical datasets including long-term ICU recordings.

Acknowledgments. This work was supported by the Institute of Information & Communications Technology Planning & Evaluation (IITP) grant funded by the Korea government (MSIT) [No. RS-2022-II220641, XVoice: Multi-Modal Voice Meta Learning], [No. RS-2022-00155915, Artificial Intelligence Convergence Innovation Human Resources Development (Inha University)].

Disclosure of Interests. The authors declare that they have no conflicts of interest.

References

1. Rubinos, C., Alkhachroum, A., Der-Nigoghossian, C., Claassen, J.: Electroencephalogram monitoring in critical care. Semin. Neurol. **40**(6), 675–680 (2020)
2. Ge, W., et al.: Deep active learning for interictal ictal injury continuum EEG patterns. J. Neurosci. Methods **351**, 108966 (2021)
3. Demir, A., Koike-Akino, T., Wang, Y., Haruna, M., Erdogmus, D.: EEG-GNN: graph neural networks for classification of electroencephalogram (EEG) signals. In: Proceedings of the Annual International Conference of the IEEE Engineering in Medicine & Biology Society (EMBC), pp. 1061–1067 (2021)
4. Du, Y., Xu, Y., Wang, X., Liu, L., Ma, P.: EEG temporal–spatial transformer for person identification. Sci. Rep. **12**(1), 14378 (2022)
5. Barnett, A.J., et al.: Improving clinician performance in classifying EEG patterns on the ictal–interictal injury continuum using interpretable machine learning. NEJM AI **1**(6) (2024)
6. Kalamangalam, G.P., Pohlmann-Eden, B.: Ictal–interictal continuum. J. Clin. Neurophysiol. **35**(4), 274–278 (2018)
7. Arnab, A., Dehghani, M., Heigold, G., Sun, C., Lučić, M., Schmid, C.: Vivit: a video vision transformer. In: Proceedings of the IEEE/CVF International Conference on Computer Vision (ICCV), pp. 6836–6846 (2021)
8. Walther, D., Viehweg, J., Haueisen, J., Mäder, P.: A systematic comparison of deep learning methods for EEG time series analysis. Front. Neuroinform. **17**, 1067095 (2023)

9. Kanamaneni, K., Venkata, R.K.: Epileptic seizures detection using deep learning techniques. NeuroQuantology **20**(10), 2939 (2022)
10. Li, D., Xu, J., Wang, J., Fang, X., Ji, Y.: A multi-scale fusion convolutional neural network based on attention mechanism for the visualization analysis of EEG signals decoding. IEEE Trans. Neural Syst. Rehabil. Eng. **28**(12), 2615–2626 (2020)
11. Bhatti, S.S., Yadav, A., Monga, M., Kumar, N.: Comparative analysis of deep learning approaches for harmful brain activity detection using EEG (2024)
12. Rosenzweig, I., et al.: Beyond the double banana: improved recognition of temporal lobe seizures in long-term EEG. J. Clin. Neurophysiol. **31**(1), 1–9 (2014)
13. Wu, W., Tan, Y.: MelicientNet: harnessing mel-spectrograms and EfficientNet architectures for predicting neurological recovery post-cardiac arrest. In: 2023 Computing in Cardiology (CinC), vol. 50, pp. 1–4 (2023)
14. Woo, S., Park, J., Lee, J.-Y., Kweon, I.S.: CBAM: convolutional block attention module. In: Proceedings of the European Conference on Computer Vision (ECCV), pp. 3–19 (2018)
15. Gong, Y., Chung, Y.-A., Glass, J.: AST: audio spectrogram transformer. In: Proceedings of Interspeech (2021)
16. Wu, H., et al.: CVT: introducing convolutions to vision transformers. In: Proceedings of the IEEE/CVF International Conference on Computer Vision (ICCV), pp. 22–31 (2021)
17. Yun, S., Han, D., Oh, S.J., Chun, S., Choe, J., Yoo, Y.: Cutmix: regularization strategy to train strong classifiers with localizable features. In: Proceedings of the IEEE/CVF International Conference on Computer Vision (ICCV), pp. 6023–6032 (2019)
18. Zhang, H.: mixup: beyond empirical risk minimization, arXiv:1710.09412 (2017)
19. Kalafatovich, J., Lee, M., Lee, S.-W.: Learning spatiotemporal graph representations for visual perception using EEG signals. IEEE Trans. Neural Syst. Rehabil. Eng. **31**, 97–108 (2022)
20. Song, Y., Zheng, Q., Liu, B., Gao, X.: EEG conformer: convolutional transformer for EEG decoding and visualization. IEEE Trans. Neural Syst. Rehabil. Eng. **31**, 710–719 (2022)
21. Jing, J., et al.: Development of expert-level classification of seizures and rhythmic and periodic patterns during EEG interpretation. Neurology **100**(17) (2023)
22. Fan, X., Xu, P., Zhao, Q., Hao, C., Zhao, Z., Wang, Z.: A domain adaption approach for EEG-based automated seizure classification with temporal-spatial-spectral attention. In: Linguraru, M.G., et al. (eds.) Proceedings of the International Conference on Medical Image Computing and Computer-Assisted Intervention (MICCAI), vol. 15005, pp. 14–24 (2024)
23. Tran, D., Wang, H., Torresani, L., Ray, J., LeCun, Y., Paluri, M.: A closer look at spatiotemporal convolutions for action recognition. In: Proceedings of the IEEE Conference on Computer Vision and Pattern Recognition (CVPR), pp. 6450–6459 (2018)
24. Jing, J., et al.: HMS - harmful brain activity classification (2024). https://kaggle.com/competitions/hms-harmful-brain-activity-classification. Kaggle
25. Holste, G., et al.: Long-tailed classification of thorax diseases on chest X-ray: a new benchmark study. In: Nguyen, H.V., Huang, S.X., Xue, Y. (eds.) Data Augmentation, Labelling, and Imperfections, vol. 13567, pp. 22–32 (2022)
26. Tilkorn, H., Mittag, G., Möller, S.: Visualising and explaining deep learning models for speech quality prediction (2021)

Priority-Aware Clinical Pathology Hierarchy Training for Multiple Instance Learning

Sungrae Hong[1], Kyungeun Kim[2], Juhyeon Kim[1], Sol Lee[1], Jisu Shin[1], Chanjae Song[1], and Mun Yong Yi[1(✉)]

[1] Graduate School of Data Science, KAIST, Daejeon, South Korea
{sr5043,wedsed123,leesol4553,jisu3389,chan4535,munyi}@kaist.ac.kr
[2] Seegene Medical Foundation, Seoul, South Korea
kekim@mf.seegene.com

Abstract. Multiple Instance Learning (MIL) is increasingly being used as a support tool within clinical settings for pathological diagnosis decisions, achieving high performance and removing the annotation burden. However, existing approaches for clinical MIL tasks have not adequately addressed the priority issues that exist in relation to pathological symptoms and diagnostic classes, causing MIL models to ignore priority among classes. To overcome this clinical limitation of MIL, we propose a new method that addresses priority issues using two hierarchies: vertical *inter-hierarchy* and horizontal *intra-hierarchy*. The proposed method aligns MIL predictions across each hierarchical level and employs an implicit feature re-usability during training to facilitate clinically more serious classes within the same level. Experiments with real-world patient data show that the proposed method effectively reduces misdiagnosis and prioritizes more important symptoms in multiclass scenarios. Further analysis verifies the efficacy of the proposed components and qualitatively confirms the MIL predictions against challenging cases with multiple symptoms.

Keywords: Multiclass Priority · Class Hierarchy · Multiple Instance Learning

1 Introduction

The exponential increase in the demand for pathological diagnoses after the COVID-19 pandemic has significantly burdened a limited number of pathological specialists [2,4]. At the same time, the deep learning (DL) community has actively pursued alleviating this workload by developing automated diagnostic models to assist pathological decision making [7]. Recently, Multiple Instance Learning (MIL), which uses only weak labels at the Whole Slide Image (WSI) level for model training, not pixel-level annotations by experts, has emerged as the golden standard in digital pathology diagnosis [22].

N. Akash et al. (Eds.): EMERGE 2025 Workshops, LNCS 16534, pp. 91–100, 2026.
https://doi.org/10.1007/978-3-032-24182-5_9

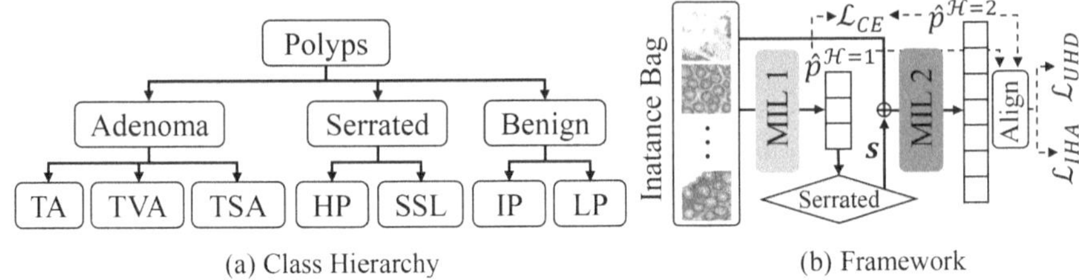

Fig. 1. (a) A diagram illustrating class relationships and hierarchy. We denote the structure from root to leaves as $\mathcal{H} = 0$ to $\mathcal{H} = 2$. (b) The proposed framework offers a two-phase design, which is trained end-to-end manner.

Although MIL offers promising results for expert assistance in clinical settings, it reveals shortcomings in multiclass scenarios, as most MIL studies have been conducted in binary settings [18,21]. Unlike binary classification, a multiclass task commonly involves a hierarchy because lower-level classes can be organized into groups of higher levels [1], potentially reflecting priorities or different clinical urgencies between those higher groups. The DL community has made several attempts to leverage hierarchy, such as loss-centric methodologies, which penalize predictions based on class relationships [1,5]. Structure-based methods try to establish these class relationships within the framework [17], graphs [3], and hyperbolic space [15]. The underlying objective of these inter-hierarchy approaches is to prevent networks from making critical fine-level errors in classification, which correspond to type II errors in medical field (*e.g.*, A model might mistake a stage of tumor, but should not confuse a cancerous cell with a normal one).

Despite previous attempts to address the hierarchy issues, the inherent properties of WSIs impose limitations on conventional multiclass hierarchy approaches. Although WSI training uses only one label, clinical inference often involves multiple symptoms, which requires pathologists to identify the most urgent problem [19,20]. As models are trained with the assumption of a strict label, they are prone to concentrate on the most probable class, rather than the most hazardous sign [10,11]. We refer to this issue, ignoring priority within the horizontal hierarchy, as an intra-hierarchy problem.

We address the hierarchy issues in multiple ways. For inter-hierarchy, we utilize a probability alignment term between each hierarchy. Concurrently, we propose a probability adjustment that allows the coarse-grained hierarchy to influence the predictions of the fine-grained hierarchy. We also present an implicit feature remix to handle the intra-hierarchy problem. Given that the input of MIL is a set of multiple instances, we implicitly train class priority by mixing instances from two samples. We have confirmed that it enables the model to focus on the more urgent class in a complex test set where two cases are mixed. The proposed framework flexibly employs MIL architectures and leverages multimodal data.

Experiments conducted on real-world clinical data show that the proposed method outperforms the extant methods while properly respecting multi-class

Table 1. Data distribution over the classes. The values in parentheses represent the number of extra test samples.

	TA	TVA	TSA	HP	SSL	IP	LP	$\sum$
Train	317	232	300	257	130	99	266	1,601
Validation	69	51	65	55	29	21	57	347
Test	164(95)	57(6)	84(18)	64(8)	84(55)	21	57	531(182)

hierarchies. Through ablation studies, we confirm the contribution of each component. Additional qualitative evaluations examine the predictions of the proposed methodology on challenging diagnostic images.

Related Work. There are several class hierarchy-aware classifiers. DeViSE [8] optimizes cosine similarity between image embeddings from pretrained visual models and label embeddings from Word2Vec [14]. Bertinetto et al. [1] introduced hierarchy-sensitive loss adaptations to reduce hierarchical distance in top-k predictions while trading off top-1 accuracy. Chang et al. [5] addressed how coarse class cross-entropy loss degrades fine-grained accuracy by partitioning the feature space to disentangle coarse and fine-grained features. Garg et al. [9] proposed a feature learning method that considers class hierarchies, using Jensen-Shannon divergence and geometric constraints to train hierarchical semantic organization. While previous studies exploited class hierarchies in a coarse-to-fine manner, the lack of explicit class priority specification within hierarchies makes hierarchical approaches worth exploring, particularly for multiclass clinical WSI settings.

2 Method

2.1 Data Description

We use 2,297 digital WSIs originated from patients in a real-world clinical setting of `Seegene Medical Foundation`[1], which comprises a total of the finest seven classes in $\mathcal{H} = 2$: tubular adenoma (TA), tubulovillous adenoma (TVA), traditional serrated adenoma (TSA), hyperplastic polyp (HP), sessile serrated lesion (SSL), inflammatory polyp (IP), and lymphoid polyp (LP). These classes are organized into three coarser categories (*i.e.*, $\mathcal{H} = 1$), as illustrated in Fig. 1(a). Among them, Adenoma is paramount due to its potential for malignant transformation. Serrated is of secondary importance, necessitating more detailed diagnosis into SSL and HP. Each WSI has a Subsite indicating specimen location: `Proximal` for near the oral cavity, `Distal` for near the anus, `UNKNOWN` otherwise. We convert it into a three-dimensional one-hot vector $\mathbf{s}$. This clinical dataset, comprising WSIs each with a single symptom, was split into training, validation,

[1] This study was performed in line with the principles of the Declaration of Helsinki. Approval was granted by the Ethics Review Board SMF-IRB-2024-007 and KH2024-059.

and test sets at a 0.7:0.15:0.15 ratio. In addition, we have incorporated an additional 182 complex samples (see Table 1), which contain two or more symptoms, into the test set, to assess the proposed method's performance in challenging real-world multi-symptom conditions.

2.2 Proposed Two-Phase Framework

Figure 1(b) shows the two-phase framework we propose in consideration of the *intra-* and *inter-* hierarchical relationships. A WSI X_i is separated into $n(X_i)$ patches $\{x_{i,1}, \cdots, x_{i,n(X_i)}\}$, and a pre-trained feature extractor outputs the corresponding instance bag $\mathcal{B}_i = \{z_{i,1}, \cdots, z_{i,n(X_i)}\}$. The $\mathcal{B}_i$ is fed into each $\mathcal{H}$ MIL, $f_{\theta_1}(\cdot)$ and $f_{\theta_2}(\cdot)$. We denote the softmax outputs of $f_{\theta_1}(\cdot)$ and $f_{\theta_2}(\cdot)$ as $\hat{p}^{\mathcal{H}=1} \in \mathbb{R}^3$ and $\hat{p}^{\mathcal{H}=2} \in \mathbb{R}^7$, respectively. Observing that pathologists closely examine the acquisition site in the diagnosis of HP and SSL, we concatenate $\mathbf{s}$ with the input to feed into $f_{\theta_2}(\cdot)$ if $\text{argmax}_c(\hat{p}^{\mathcal{H}=1})$ is Serrated. Consequently, each hierarchy MIL is trained in an end-to-end manner with the proposed framework using the following cross-entropy term:

$$\mathcal{L}_{CE} = -\frac{1}{2} \sum_{h \in \mathcal{H}} \sum_{c \in \mathcal{C}^{\mathcal{H}=h}} y_c^{\mathcal{H}=h} \log(\hat{p}_c^{\mathcal{H}=h}) \tag{1}$$

where $\mathcal{C}^{\mathcal{H}}$ indicates the classes that are allocated in $\mathcal{H}$.

2.3 Inter-hierarchy Alignment

Although hierarchical MILs predict a different number of classes, they share the same input. That is, given that both MILs evaluate the same samples, the lower-level probability distribution, aggregated to match the higher-level classes, should ideally match the higher-level probability distribution. Inspired by this motivation and [9], we enforce $\hat{p}^{\mathcal{H}=1}$ and $\hat{p}^{\mathcal{H}=2}$ to be aligned:

$$\mathcal{L}_{IHA} = \text{JS}(\hat{p}^{\mathcal{H}=1} || \dot{p}^{\mathcal{H}=1}) = \frac{1}{2}\left(\text{KL}(\hat{p}^{\mathcal{H}=1} || m) + \text{KL}(\dot{p}^{\mathcal{H}=1} || m)\right) \tag{2}$$

where $m = \frac{1}{2} \times (\hat{p}^{\mathcal{H}=1} + \dot{p}^{\mathcal{H}=1})$. JS and KL denote Jensen-Shannon Divergence and Kullback-Leibler Divergence, respectively. We perform the following operation to obtain the average distribution $m \in \mathbb{R}^3$ and the aligned probability $\dot{p}^{\mathcal{H}=1} \in \mathbb{R}^3$ from $\mathcal{H} = 2$ to $\mathcal{H} = 1$:

$$\dot{p}_c^{\mathcal{H}=1} = \sum_{c' \subset c} \hat{p}_{c'}^{\mathcal{H}=2}, \text{ where } c \in \mathcal{C}^{\mathcal{H}=1} \text{ and } c' \in \mathcal{C}^{\mathcal{H}=2}. \tag{3}$$

2.4 Upper-Hierarchy-Dependent Probability

Classifying the three classes of $\mathcal{H} = 1$ is a simpler task than the seven classes of $\mathcal{H} = 2$. In other words, if $f_{\theta_1}(\cdot)$ and $f_{\theta_2}(\cdot)$ refer to each other, it is reasonable to do so from the coarse to the fine level. Therefore, we adjust the probabilities

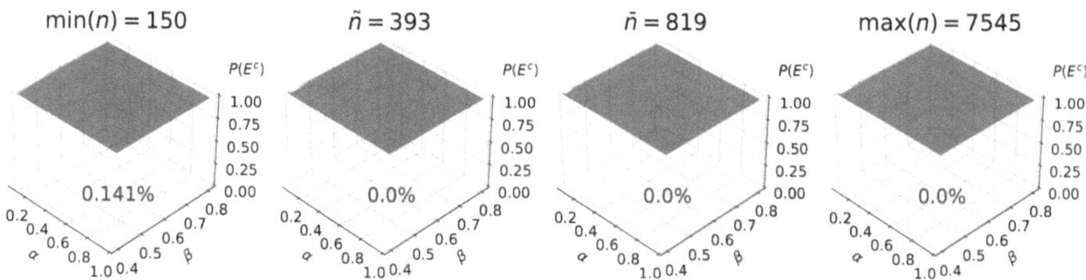

Fig. 2. Visualization of the probability of event E not occurring (Eq. 5). $P(E^c)$ is visualized for the median, average, and maximum counts of $n = |\mathcal{B}_i|$. In each plot, the blue percentage indicates the proportion of cases with a probability of 99% or less out of feasible events.

$\hat{p}^{\mathcal{H}=2}$ of $f_{\theta_2}(\cdot)$, so that it aligns with the predictions of the $f_{\theta_1}(\cdot)$ while also allowing for some dependence:

$$\mathcal{L}_{UHD} = \mathrm{KL}(||\tilde{p}^{\mathcal{H}=2}||_1||y^{\mathcal{H}=2})$$
$$\text{, where } \tilde{p}_c^{\mathcal{H}=2} = \begin{cases} \hat{p}_c^{\mathcal{H}=2} \times \hat{p}_{c'}^{\mathcal{H}=1} & \text{, if } c \subset c' \\ \hat{p}_c^{\mathcal{H}=2} & \text{, otherwise.} \end{cases} \tag{4}$$

2.5 Implicit Feature Remix for Intra-Hierarchy

We still have the second component of the class hierarchy: Intra-hierarchy. Given that a $\mathcal{B}$ is a collection of multiple instances, a random proportion $\beta \sim \mathrm{Uniform}(0.4, 0.8)$ of instances is sampled from $\mathcal{B}_i$ and mixed into the $1-\beta$ proportion of $\mathcal{B}_j$ to synthesize bag $\mathcal{B}_{i+j}$, where $\mathcal{B}_i$ has higher priority than $\mathcal{B}_j$ within the same $\mathcal{H}$ (*e.g.*, TA and LP). We perform feature remixing only when $\mathcal{B}_i$ has at least 150 instances to create a distinguishable synthesized sample. Here, a valid concern is the possibility that the following event E occurs: $E = \{$*no crucial instance for diagnosis from* $\mathcal{B}_i$ *are mixed into* $\mathcal{B}_{i+j}\}$. However, contrary to our concerns, if we assume $\mathcal{B}_i$ contains a proportion of $\alpha \geq 0.05$ instances exhibiting symptoms, then event E is rarely to occur (*i.e.*, complementary set E^c) as depicted in following Eq. 5 and its visualization Fig. 2:

$$P(E^c) = \begin{cases} 1 - \frac{{}_{(n-n\alpha)}C_{n\beta}}{{}_{n}C_{n\beta}} & \text{, if } \alpha + \beta < 1 \\ 1 & \text{, if } \alpha + \beta \geq 1. \end{cases} \tag{5}$$

Furthermore, we introduce label softening to utilize the benefits of label softening [6], where k-th dimension of the smoothed label vector $y_{i+j}^{\mathcal{H}}$ is defined as:

Table 2. The performance comparisons of alternative hierarchy-aware methods. The values in parentheses indicate standard deviation.

TransMIL [18]						
Method	$\mathcal{H}=1$			$\mathcal{H}=2$		
	Accuracy	AUROC	Recall	Accuracy	AUROC	Recall
CE	-	-	-	0.866(0.008)	0.987(0.001)	0.933(0.020)
Weighted CE (5:3:2)	-	-	-	0.870(0.012)	0.987(0.001)	0.933(0.020)
Weighted CE (7:2:1)	-	-	-	0.851(0.011)	0.986(0.002)	0.916(0.027)
HXE ($\alpha=0.1$) [1]	0.916(0.009)	0.985(0.002)	0.908(0.013)	0.876(0.017)	0.987(0.002)	0.948(0.008)
HXE ($\alpha=0.3$) [1]	0.912(0.010)	0.986(0.002)	**0.937(0.027)**	0.875(0.007)	0.988(0.001)	0.941(0.017)
Soft Labels ($\beta=5$) [1]	0.908(0.009)	0.982(0.004)	0.914(0.012)	0.882(0.012)	0.985(0.002)	0.953(0.012)
Soft Labels ($\beta=10$) [1]	0.918(0.014)	0.981(0.011)	0.929(0.022)	0.868(0.009)	0.982(0.002)	0.933(0.017)
Chang et al. [5]	0.920(0.009)	0.981(0.003)	0.924(0.009)	0.872(0.007)	0.985(0.003)	0.941(0.013)
HAF [9]	0.865(0.045)	0.960(0.003)	0.910(0.042)	0.869(0.015)	0.986(0.002)	0.940(0.022)
Ours	**0.922(0.009)**	**0.989(0.001)**	0.927(0.029)	**0.898(0.006)**	**0.990(0.002)**	**0.972(0.008)**
DTFD-MIL [21]						
CE	-	-	-	0.860(0.014)	0.986(0.002)	0.918(0.016)
Weighted CE (5:3:2)	-	-	-	0.871(0.012)	0.987(0.001)	0.933(0.020)
Weighted CE (7:2:1)	-	-	-	0.850(0.019)	0.984(0.002)	0.896(0.014)
HXE ($\alpha=0.1$) [1]	0.922(0.023)	0.985(0.002)	0.911(0.053)	0.875(0.003)	0.987(0.001)	0.934(0.012)
HXE ($\alpha=0.3$) [1]	0.926(0.009)	0.987(0.001)	0.924(0.020)	0.863(0.003)	0.987(0.001)	0.924(0.006)
Soft Labels ($\beta=5$) [1]	0.923(0.011)	0.986(0.003)	0.925(0.015)	0.874(0.007)	0.980(0.002)	0.927(0.010)
Soft Labels ($\beta=10$) [1]	0.915(0.010)	0.983(0.004)	0.916(0.022)	0.866(0.008)	0.984(0.002)	0.930(0.018)
Chang et al. [5]	0.941(0.008)	0.987(0.002)	0.944(0.027)	0.879(0.016)	0.987(0.004)	0.947(0.016)
HAF [9]	0.894(0.023)	0.976(0.006)	0.865(0.042)	0.862(0.012)	0.986(0.003)	0.916(0.020)
Ours	**0.948(0.007)**	**0.991(0.001)**	**0.955(0.013)**	**0.892(0.014)**	**0.991(0.001)**	**0.970(0.010)**

$$y^{\mathcal{H}}_{i+j,k} = \begin{cases} \tilde{r}_k/(\tilde{r}_i+\tilde{r}_j), \text{ if } k \in \{i,j\} \\ 0 \quad\quad\quad\quad , \text{ otherwise.} \end{cases}$$
$$, \text{ where } \begin{cases} \tilde{r}_i = r^{1/\tau} \\ \tilde{r}_j = (1-r)^{\tau} \end{cases} \text{ and } r = \frac{\beta \times |\mathcal{B}_i|}{\beta \times |\mathcal{B}_i| + (1-\beta)\times|\mathcal{B}_j|} \tag{6}$$

where τ is the smoothing factor. The condition for $\bar{r}_i$ and $\bar{r}_j$ is designed to make the class of $\mathcal{B}_i$ dominant in $y^{\mathcal{H}}_{i+j}$.

The proposed hierarchical MIL framework is trained by the term $\mathcal{L} = \mathcal{L}_{CE} + \mathcal{L}_{IHA} + \mathcal{L}_{UHD}$.

3 Experiment

3.1 Implementation Details

MIL Architectures. We utilize two state-of-the-art MIL architectures: TransMIL [18] and DTFD MIL [21]. TransMIL optimizes computation while capturing more advanced inter-instance relationships. DTFD-MIL conducts double-tier distillation by resampling the input into pseudo-bags. For DTDF-MIL, we adopt Aggregated Feature Selection, which typically yields superior performance.

Training Settings. We set the τ as 15. We selected $\times$256 size patches from the 1MPP of WSIs using the Otsu algorithm [16], then transformed them into

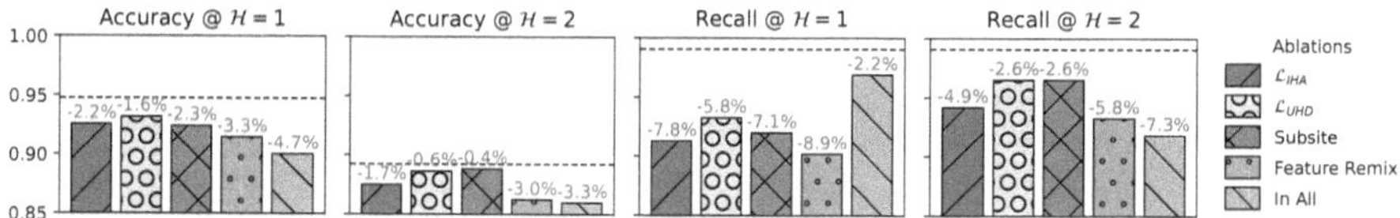

Fig. 3. Ablation results on the core components of the proposed method using DTFD-MIL. Dashed lines indicate the fully equipped model's performance.

individual instances with a pre-trained feature extractor [12]. We trained the model using Adam optimizer [13] with betas of $(0.9, 0.999)$ and a learning rate of $1e-4$. All experiments were carried out with fixed seeds on a single NVIDIA® A6000 with 48 GB of memory.

Comparison Methods. We set cross-entropy (CE) and weighted CE, which explicitly trains for the importance of classes, as the baseline. Hierarchical CE (HXE) and soft labels [1], Chang et al. [5], and hierarchy-aware feature (HAF) [9] were selected as comparison methods that can handle coarse-to-fine hierarchy. For fair comparisons, we repeated all experiments with the optimized hyper-parameters for each method, reporting the mean and standard deviation.

Evaluation Metrics. We evaluate the performance at each $\mathcal{H}$ with Accuracy, AUROC, and Recall scores.

In particular, the recall measure used here is based on a binary metric, where the positive class is defined as Adenoma or any of its subclasses.

3.2 Quantitative Results

Table 2 presents the results of running various hierarchy-aware methods against the test data. Applying weighted CE with 5:3:2 weights improves the baseline in both MIL structures. However, it also shows that excessively high weights for certain classes can reverse this gain, making performance worse than the baseline, highlighting that methods requiring explicit parameterization necessitate domain expertise and considerable empirical search.

Moreover, HXE [1] had difficulty leveraging its advantages in the minimal depth hierarchy because its conditional term operates with limited information, which hinders the differentiation of importance of the class. Consistent performance gains are observed across all comparison groups with the weak soft-labels [1] (*i.e.*, $\beta = 5$). The HAF [9] results reveal that hierarchical feature alignment is not critical for MIL. This phenomenon can be attributed to the representational disparity: linear networks exhibit limited interaction while attention-based MIL captures nuanced feature correlations, which are not adaptable across the hierarchies. Upon the results of Chang et al. [5], it shows remarkable performance at $\mathcal{H} = 1$ compared to other methods, due to training that emphasized coarser information through initial epochs. Finally, our proposed approach yielded superior performance compared to other methods, without exception. Not only did it ensure high accuracy, but also showed the lowest type

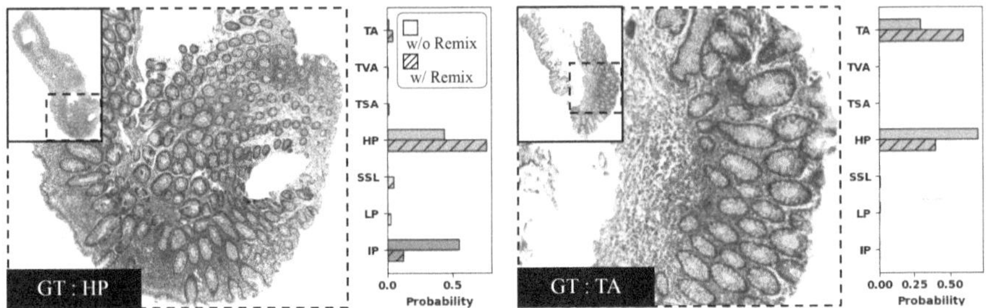

Fig. 4. Quantitative investigation into cases with mixed symptoms. We plot the $\hat{p}^{\mathcal{H}=2}$ of models trained with feature remixed samples against those of models trained without, shown with the corresponding WSIs.

II error rates, which is critical in medical domain. The findings indicate that our approach provides a suitable solution for real-world clinical WSIs, considering their vertical inter-class hierarchy and diagnostic priority at the same level.

3.3 Further Analysis

Ablation Study. We have conducted an ablation study to understand each component's effect on performance. Results of removing $\mathcal{L}_{IHA}$, $\mathcal{L}_{UHD}$, subsite $\mathbf{s}$, feature remix, and all components are shown in Fig. 3. Each removal caused performance degradation, with excluding all components showing the worst results. Removing subsite at $\mathcal{H} = 2$ also affected precision at $\mathcal{H} = 1$, indicating probability alignment impacts $\mathcal{H} = 1$ performance. Feature remix ablation resulted in the most substantial degradation, highlighting its importance for WSIs with multiple symptoms. Moreover, regarding the feature remix component, the concurrent increase in both recall and accuracy suggests that the improved recall is derived from precise diagnoses, not simply over-predicting positive cases.

Analysis on Intra-Hierarchy. To understand how the model performs against challenging cases, we have examined whether the model prioritizes the most urgent class when two or more cases are mixed within a WSI. The left tissue in Fig. 4 presents an HP with substantial IP mixture. Without intra-hierarchy training, the MIL model predicts IP with greater confidence than HP, simply due to the symptom area. In contrast, a model that implicitly learns the diagnostic precedence of HP over IP predicts the case with the more serious diagnosis. The tissue on the right is a sample that pathologists diagnose as TA, but previous MIL approaches classified it as HP. Although a small area of TA is observed in the magnified view, it is expected to have a higher probability because it is more urgent than HP. Implicit feature remix prioritizes the class with higher precedence when multiple classes are present in an instance bag.

4 Conclusion

Our research aims to solve the constraints that currently impede the successful implementation of multiclass WSI MIL in real-world clinical settings. With the formulation of the class hierarchy in two alternative ways, our proposed method offers key components effective for each. Inter-hierarchy alignment of predictions across the vertical hierarchy contributes to improved performance. The predictions of the fine-grained hierarchy are influenced by the coarse-grained hierarchy, thus having fine probabilities adjusted to ensure consistency with the coarse. Implicit feature remix allows the model to understand diagnostic urgency in mixed-symptom inference environments, relying solely on a weak label. The results of the experiment have shown that the feature remix improved the quantitative performance and allowed it to focus on more prioritized diagnoses. Furthermore, we have explored the applicability of the class hierarchy, a novel concept in MIL, by comparing it with various methods. Our proposed method mitigates the challenges of multiclass MIL diagnosis of previous approaches, broadening its applicability to practical use in clinical settings.

Acknowledgment. This research was supported by the Seegene Medical Foundation, South Korea, under the project "Development of a Multimodal Artificial Intelligence-Based Computer-Aided Diagnosis System for Gastrointestinal Endoscopic Biopsies" (Grant Number: G01240151).

Disclosure of Interests. The authors have no competing interests to declare that are relevant to the content of this article.

References

1. Bertinetto, L., Mueller, R., Tertikas, K., Samangooei, S., Lord, N.A.: Making better mistakes: leveraging class hierarchies with deep networks. In: Proceedings of the IEEE/CVF Conference on Computer Vision and Pattern Recognition, pp. 12506–12515 (2020)
2. Bray, F., Laversanne, M., Weiderpass, E., Soerjomataram, I.: The ever-increasing importance of cancer as a leading cause of premature death worldwide. Cancer **127**(16), 3029–3030 (2021)
3. Brust, C.A., Denzler, J.: Integrating domain knowledge: using hierarchies to improve deep classifiers. In: Asian Conference on Pattern Recognition, pp. 3–16. Springer (2019)
4. Bychkov, A., Schubert, M.: Constant demand, patchy supply. Pathologist **88**, 18–27 (2023)
5. Chang, D., Pang, K., Zheng, Y., Ma, Z., Song, Y.Z., Guo, J.: Your "flamingo" is my "bird": fine-grained, or not. In: Proceedings of the IEEE/CVF Conference on Computer Vision and Pattern Recognition, pp. 11476–11485 (2021)
6. Chen, B., Ziyin, L., Wang, Z., Liang, P.P.: An investigation of how label smoothing affects generalization. arXiv preprint arXiv:2010.12648 (2020)
7. Echle, A., Rindtorff, N.T., Brinker, T.J., Luedde, T., Pearson, A.T., Kather, J.N.: Deep learning in cancer pathology: a new generation of clinical biomarkers. Br. J. Cancer **124**(4), 686–696 (2021)

8. Frome, A., et al.: Devise: a deep visual-semantic embedding model. In: Advances in Neural Information Processing Systems, vol. 26 (2013)
9. Garg, A., Sani, D., Anand, S.: Learning hierarchy aware features for reducing mistake severity. In: European Conference on Computer Vision, pp. 252–267. Springer (2022)
10. Goyal, M., Yap, M.H., Hassanpour, S.: Multi-class semantic segmentation of skin lesions via fully convolutional networks. arXiv preprint arXiv:1711.10449 (2017)
11. Guo, C., Pleiss, G., Sun, Y., Weinberger, K.Q.: On calibration of modern neural networks. In: International Conference on Machine Learning, pp. 1321–1330. PMLR (2017)
12. Kang, M., Song, H., Park, S., Yoo, D., Pereira, S.: Benchmarking self-supervised learning on diverse pathology datasets. In: Proceedings of the IEEE/CVF Conference on Computer Vision and Pattern Recognition, pp. 3344–3354 (2023)
13. Kingma, D.P.: Adam: a method for stochastic optimization. arXiv preprint arXiv:1412.6980 (2014)
14. Mikolov, T., Chen, K., Corrado, G., Dean, J.: Efficient estimation of word representations in vector space. arXiv preprint arXiv:1301.3781 (2013)
15. Nickel, M., Kiela, D.: Poincaré embeddings for learning hierarchical representations. In: Advances in Neural Information Processing Systems, vol. 30 (2017)
16. Otsu, N., et al.: A threshold selection method from gray-level histograms. Automatica **11**(285–296), 23–27 (1975)
17. Redmon, J., Farhadi, A.: Yolo9000: better, faster, stronger. In: Proceedings of the IEEE Conference on Computer Vision and Pattern Recognition, pp. 7263–7271 (2017)
18. Shao, Z., Bian, H., Chen, Y., Wang, Y., Zhang, J., Ji, X., et al.: Transmil: transformer based correlated multiple instance learning for whole slide image classification. Adv. Neural. Inf. Process. Syst. **34**, 2136–2147 (2021)
19. Williams, B.J., Bottoms, D., Treanor, D.: Future-proofing pathology: the case for clinical adoption of digital pathology. J. Clin. Pathol. **70**(12), 1010–1018 (2017)
20. Wong, A.N.N., et al.: Current developments of artificial intelligence in digital pathology and its future clinical applications in gastrointestinal cancers. Cancers **14**(15), 3780 (2022)
21. Zhang, H., et al.: DTFD-MIL: double-tier feature distillation multiple instance learning for histopathology whole slide image classification. In: Proceedings of the IEEE/CVF Conference on Computer Vision and Pattern Recognition, pp. 18802–18812 (2022)
22. Zhang, Y., Gao, Z., He, K., Li, C., Mao, R.: From patches to WSIs: a systematic review of deep multiple instance learning in computational pathology. Inf. Fusion 103027 (2025)

Poster Presentations

Invisible Yet Detected: PelFANet with Attention-Guided Anatomical Fusion for Pelvic Fracture Diagnosis

Siam Tahsin Bhuiyan[1(✉)], Rashedur Rahman[1], Sefatul Wasi[1], Naomi Yagi[2], Syoji Kobashi[3], Ashraful Islam[1], and Saadia Binte Alam[1]

[1] Independent University, Dhaka, Bangladesh
ciamtbhuiyan@gmail.com
[2] Advanced Medical Engineering Research Institute, University of Hyogo, Kobe, Japan
[3] Graduate School of Engineering, University of Hyogo, Kobe, Japan

Abstract. Pelvic fractures pose significant diagnostic challenges, particularly in cases where fracture signs are subtle or invisible on standard radiographs. To address this, we introduce PelFANet, a dual-stream attention network that fuses raw pelvic X-rays with segmented bone images to improve fracture classification. The network employs Fused Attention Blocks (FABlocks) to iteratively exchange and refine features from both inputs, capturing global context and localized anatomical detail. Trained in a two-stage pipeline with a segmentation-guided approach, PelFANet demonstrates superior performance over conventional methods. On the AMERI dataset, it achieves 88.68% accuracy and 0.9334 AUC on visible fractures, while generalizing effectively to invisible fracture cases with 82.29% accuracy and 0.8688 AUC, despite not being trained on them. These results highlight the clinical potential of anatomy-aware dual-input architectures for robust fracture detection, especially in scenarios with subtle radiographic presentations.

Keywords: PelFANet · Invisible Fracture Detection · Anatomy-Guided Attention · Pelvic X-ray Classification

1 Introduction

Pelvic fractures are among the most critical injuries in emergency medicine, typically caused by high-energy trauma such as motor vehicle accidents or falls [1]. Due to the pelvis's anatomical complexity and its role in protecting vital organs and blood vessels, such fractures can lead to severe complications, including hemorrhage and multi-organ damage [2]. In-hospital mortality rates range from 5% to 20%, influenced by fracture severity, hemorrhagic shock, and associated injuries [3, 4].

Diagnosis relies heavily on radiographic evaluation and clinician expertise [5], which poses challenges in trauma settings. Subtle or complex fractures are often missed, even by skilled radiologists [6]. In high-pressure environments, diagnostic errors are common,

N. Akash et al. (Eds.): EMERGE 2025 Workshops, LNCS 16534, pp. 103–113, 2026.
https://doi.org/10.1007/978-3-032-24182-5_10

with up to 20% of pelvic fractures initially overlooked in trauma centers [7], resulting in delayed treatment, worsening injuries, and increased mortality [8]. Rapid and accurate detection is thus essential.

Recent studies have demonstrated strong performance in pelvic and femur fracture detection using deep learning frameworks, achieving accuracies in the range of 80–98% [9, 10]. Segmentation-guided classification is a powerful method that enhances classification accuracy by localizing specific regions of interest before feature extraction and prediction. In the context of medical imaging, this technique is especially useful for focusing on diagnostically relevant anatomical structures while ignoring irrelevant background noise. Segmentation-guided classification has proven effective across various domains, including colorectal cancer, liver cancer, and pneumonia, by improving diagnostic focus and reducing false negatives [11–15]. A recent study [16] proposed the APEx framework, leveraging a query-based segmentation transformer to jointly model anatomical and pathological features, resulting in improved segmentation performance on FDG-PET-CT and chest X-ray datasets. These methods are particularly valuable in low-contrast or cluttered imaging scenarios common issues in pelvic X-rays where global analysis may be insufficient for accurate fracture detection.

Recent studies have shown the effectiveness of segmentation-guided pelvic fracture classification. [17] Reported 96.32% DSC and 98.03% accuracy using Swin U-Net, while [18] achieved 0.96–0.97 DSC and 69–88% classification accuracy across pelvic ring fracture types using an Association for Osteosynthesis (AO) Foundation and Orthopedic Trauma Association (OTA) (AO/OTA)-guided system.

However, fracture diagnosis in pelvic radiographs can benefit significantly from contextual background information beyond the bone boundaries. While some fractures show clear cortical disruptions, others present subtle signs such as abnormal alignment, joint spacing, or limb asymmetry indicators that may lie outside the segmented bone region. Studies have shown that non-local cues like limb rotation, joint dislocation, or pubic symphysis widening can suggest fractures even in the absence of visible cortical breaks [19, 20]. Segmenting out only the bone often removes these diagnostic cues, whereas raw pelvic X-rays preserve the full anatomical context, including soft tissue and alignment, which can be crucial for detecting such subtle injuries.

This is particularly relevant in cases of invisible fractures, pelvic X-ray (PXR) images without obvious fracture signs but confirmed via 3D-CT imaging. As demonstrated in recent work, these cases are challenging for existing deep learning methods [21]. Our work addresses this by leveraging both raw and segmented inputs to retain global structure and enhance diagnostic robustness.

To address the limitations of relying solely on either segmentation or raw image analysis, we propose PelFANet, a Pelvic Fused Attention Network that integrates both segmented bone structures and raw pelvic X-rays through a dual-stream attention-guided fusion architecture. By combining localized anatomical detail with full-field context, PelFANet is designed to detect both overt and subtle fracture cues. The streams are fused using Convolutional Block Attention Module (CBAM)-based attention [22], allowing the model to learn feature combinations from both inputs that contribute to improved classification. PelFANet outperforms existing approaches by accurately detecting both visible fractures and invisible fractures, by leveraging subtle contextual and anatomical cues indicative of underlying injury.

2 Methodology

2.1 Overview

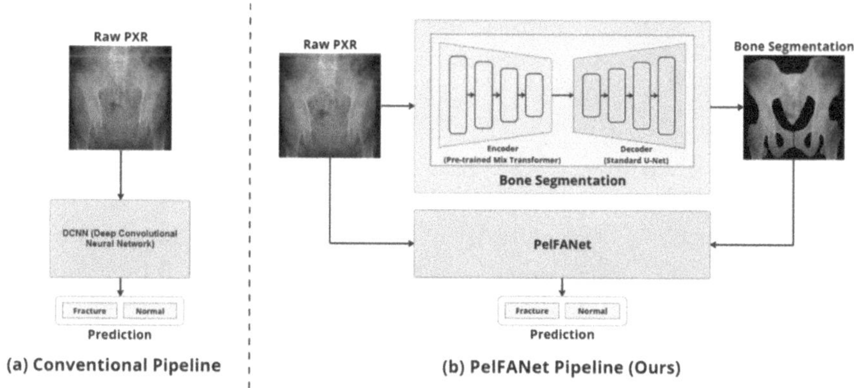

Fig. 1. (a) Single-stream baseline using raw PXR for direct fracture prediction. (b) Proposed PelFANet pipeline combining raw PXR and segmented bone via a dual-stream attention network.

Our framework consists of a two-stage pipeline: a segmentation model generates segmented bones from raw pelvic X-rays, which are then combined with the original PXRs and fed into PelFANet, a dual-stream network with attention-based fusion. This setup integrates anatomical detail with global context for improved fracture detection illustrated in Fig. 1.

2.2 Bone Segmentation

To incorporate anatomical context into the classification process, we first generate segmented bones using a U-Net with a Mix Transformer B0 encoder [23–25]. This hybrid architecture combines U-Net's spatial accuracy with the transformer's global context modeling, enabling precise delineation of pelvic bones. The implementation follows the [25] segmentation library, which provides modular support for both the U-Net structure and transformer-based encoders.

Considering the full Pelvic region as a single class we train a one-class segmentation model. Once trained, the model infers bone masks, which are cropped to produce the segmented bones used as the second input to PelFANet, guiding fracture classification with structure-aware features.

2.3 PelFANet

Input. PelFANet uses a dual-input design, combining each raw pelvic X-ray with its corresponding bone segmentation. Both inputs are resized into a 224 × 224 image, then passed into two streams for separate processing. This setup enables the network to leverage both structural and contextual cues for accurate fracture classification.

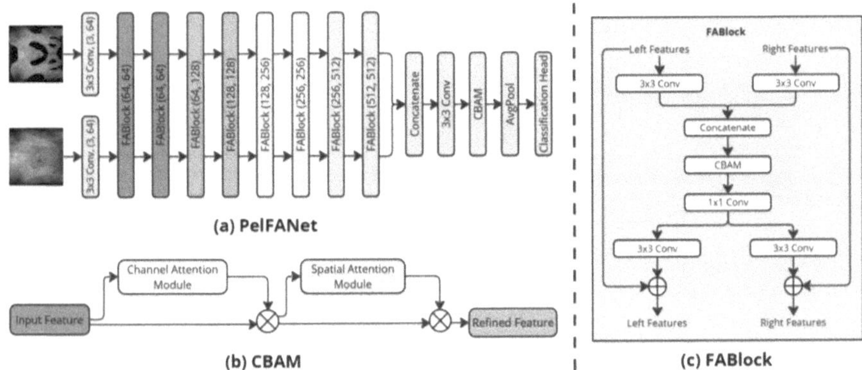

Fig. 2. (a) PelFANet architecture: a dual-stream attention network that processes raw PXRs and bone segmentations via parallel branches, fused using stacked Fused Attention Blocks (FABlock). (b) Structure of the CBAM attention module. (c) FABlock design: stream-specific convolution, CBAM-based fusion, and residual redistribution into both branches.

Network Architecture. PelFANet is a dual-stream convolutional architecture specifically designed to fuse global context from raw pelvic X-rays and fine-grained anatomical structure from bone segmentations. The network is composed of three main stages: parallel feature extraction, attention-guided fusion through stacked Fused Attention Blocks (FABlock), and final aggregation and classification.

In the initial stage, the raw pelvic X-ray and its corresponding bone segmentation are passed through two independent convolutional branches. Each stream begins with a 3 × 3 convolution layer, followed by batch normalization, ReLU activation, and max pooling. These parallel branches extract low-level features specific to the raw and segmented modalities.

The core of the network consists of eight FABlocks. At each FABlock, the feature maps from the left and right branches are independently processed, concatenated, and passed through a CBAM to generate attention-refined fused features. These fused features are then projected via a 1 × 1 convolution and split back into the two original streams. Residual connections and convolutional layers further refine the separated features before concatenation. This repeated fusion and redistribution mechanism allows the model to dynamically integrate complementary features across modalities while maintaining stream-specific information.

Following the FABlocks, the fused features undergo global attention refinement and pooling before final classification through a fully connected layer.

This architecture illustrated in Fig. 2, enables the network to reason jointly over global cues and localized bone structures, improving its ability to detect subtle or complex fracture patterns that may not be captured by single-source models.

FABlock. The FABlock is the core unit of PelFANet, enabling interactive feature refinement between the raw pelvic X-ray stream and the bone segmentation stream. Let the input feature maps from these two streams be $F_1 \in \mathbb{R}^{C \times H \times W}$ and $F_2 \in \mathbb{R}^{C \times H \times W}$, where C, H, W represent the number of channels, height, and width, respectively.

First, each input is passed through a stream-specific convolution:

$$F_1' = f_{3\times3}(F_1), F_2' = f_{3\times3}(F_2) \tag{1}$$

The outputs are concatenated channel-wise, where $F_{cat} \in \mathbb{R}^{2C \times H \times W}$:

$$F_{cat} = Concat\left(F_1', F_2'\right) \tag{2}$$

This combined feature map is refined using the CBAM. CBAM sequentially applies channel and spatial attention to highlight informative features. The CBAM-refined fused feature map is denoted as:

$$CFA = f_{1\times1}(CBAM\,(F_{cat})) \tag{3}$$

This output, CFA (Combined Feature with Attention), is then used to update the original streams using additional convolution and residual addition:

$$NF_1 = F_1 + f_{3\times3}(CFA), NF_2 = F_2 + f_{3\times3}(CFA) \tag{4}$$

where NF_1 and NF_2 are the updated feature maps for the raw X-ray and segmentation streams, respectively. These outputs are then forwarded to the next FABlock, enabling progressive cross-stream refinement with attention.

Final Feature Aggregation and Classification. The fused feature map from the final FABlock is passed through a 3×3 convolution followed by CBAM attention, batch normalization, and ReLU activation. Global features are then extracted using adaptive average pooling and flattened into a 1024-dimensional vector. This vector is passed through a fully connected layer to produce the final classification output, enabling prediction of fracture presence based on the combined raw and anatomical information.

3 Experiments

3.1 Datasets

AMERI Dataset. The Visible Fracture subset (VIS) of the AMERI PXR dataset consists of 228 pelvic X-ray images, including 168 fracture cases and 60 normal cases. These were selected from a larger set of 481 pelvic X-rays collected from 315 subjects at Steel Memorial Hirohata Hospital in Japan between April 2013 and August 2019. All fracture cases were confirmed by experienced radiologists. To ensure data quality, cases with implants or incomplete pelvic coverage were excluded.

We also curated a dedicated Invisible Fracture subset (INVIS) comprising 23 fracture and 12 normal cases. These fractures are not visible in X-rays but were confirmed through corresponding 3D-CT scans, providing a challenging benchmark for evaluating the model's ability to detect subtle and context-dependent fractures.

COVID QU-Ex Dataset. We utilize the COVID-QU-Ex dataset for pretraining, which comprises 33,920 chest X-ray (CXR) images categorized into three classes: COVID-19 (11,956), Non-COVID infections such as viral or bacterial pneumonia (11,263), and Normal (10,701) [26–30]. Crucially, the dataset provides ground-truth lung masks for all images, making it one of the largest public sets. This paired data enabled effective pretraining before fine-tuning on pelvic X-rays.

3.2 Segmentation Training and Setup

We trained a U-Net with Mix Transformer B0 encoder (pretrained on ImageNet) on the AMERI dataset using 2-fold cross-validation (228 images split equally, resized to 224 × 224). Data augmentation included geometric (ShiftScaleRotate, Perspective, Crop, Padding), intensity (CLAHE, Brightness-Contrast, Gamma), and texture/color (Sharpening, Blurring, Motion Blur, HSV) applied probabilistically. The binary segmentation model employed a sigmoid activation in the final layer and was optimized using Dice Loss. It was trained for 300 epochs with the Adam optimizer (initial learning rate (LR) of $2 \times 10^{-}4$), a cosine annealing scheduler (minimum LR $1 \times 10^{-}5$, cycle length of 50), and a batch size of 25.

3.3 PelFANet Training and Setup

The model was pretrained on the COVID-QU-Ex dataset because it exposed the network to a wide range of anatomical structures and radiographic variations, reducing the likelihood of over-specialization to the training set.

The dataset was split into 80% training and 20% testing, with 20% of the training set used for validation. Each image was augmented four times using random rotation (within 25°), shearing (within 10%), horizontal flipping, and translation (within 10%), expanding the training set to 108,575 images.

Pretraining was conducted using CrossEntropyLoss with a Stochastic Gradient Descent (SGD) optimizer (LR = 0.0001) and a StepLR scheduler that reduced the learning rate by a factor of 0.1 every 10 epochs. The model was trained for 100 epochs with a batch size of 64.

For fine-tuning, a reshuffled 5-fold cross-validation was applied to the VIS subset. To address class imbalance, each fracture case was augmented into 2 variants and each normal case into 6, using the same augmentation strategy. The final classification layer was changed from three to two outputs, and the entire model was retrained using the same loss, optimizer, and scheduler. Fine-tuning ran for 30 epochs with a batch size of 8.

4 Result

4.1 Segmentation Performance

The bone segmentation model was evaluated using Intersection over Union (IoU) and Dice Score. The model achieved high segmentation accuracy across both folds.

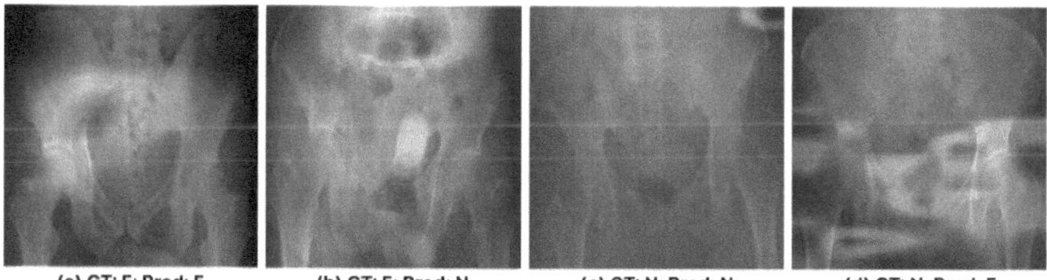

Fig. 3. Grad-CAM visualizations from PelFANet for different prediction scenarios, where GT stands for Ground Truth, F denotes Fracture and N denotes Normal. Heatmaps indicate regions influencing the model's decision.

An average IoU 90.28% and an average Dice Score of 92.78%, these results confirm the effectiveness of our segmentation setup, providing reliable and accurate anatomical masks that serve as critical inputs to the PelFANet classifier.

4.2 PelFANet Classification Performance

Following segmentation, the PelFANet architecture processes both the raw PXR and the segmentation mask to perform fracture classification. Performance metrics, averaged across the 5-fold setup along with the fold variance, are shown in Table 1. On the VIS subset, PelFANet achieved an accuracy of 88.68% (±0.11%), precision of 92.49% (±0.09%), recall of 92.21% (±0.17%), and an AUC of 0.9334 (±0.10). While the model demonstrates strong sensitivity with high recall, the specificity of 78.33% (±1.27%) indicates a moderate rate of false positives, reflecting a trade-off between detecting fractures and avoiding misclassification of normal cases. Most importantly, PelFANet was evaluated on the challenging INVIS subset, where fractures are not visible in the pelvic X-rays. Although trained exclusively on visible fracture cases, the model generalized well to this difficult set, achieving 82.29% (±0.01%) accuracy, 88.36% (±0.07%) precision, 84.35% (±0.07%) recall, 78.33% (±0.44%) specificity, and an AUC of 0.8688 (±0.04). The low variance values across metrics indicate consistent performance, though specificity shows slightly higher variance on the VIS subset, reflecting some variability in detecting fractures across folds. These results suggest that PelFANet captures deeper, more abstract fracture features by effectively integrating both global context and localized anatomical information.

Combining both raw PXR images and bone segmentation masks with attention mechanisms likely contributed to this improved performance. The bone segmentations not only guide the model to focus on diagnostically important regions but also retain spatial

Table 1. PelFANet Performance on Visible (VIS) and Invisible (INVIS) Subsets

Fracture Type	Accuracy (Variance)	Precision (Variance)	Recall (Variance)	Specificity (Variance)	F1 Score (Variance)	AUC (Variance)
VIS	88.68% (0.11%)	92.49% (0.09%)	92.21% (0.17%)	78.33% (1.27%)	84.71% (0.46%)	0.9334 (0.10)
INVIS	82.29% (0.01%)	88.36% (0.07%)	84.35% (0.07%)	78.33% (0.44%)	81.23% (0.06%)	0.8688 (0.04)

correspondence with the raw input, which is especially useful for subtle or non-local signs of fracture. As illustrated in Fig. 3, Gradient-weighted Class Activation Mapping (Grad-CAM) visualizations reveal that correctly classified fracture cases exhibit focused activation on relevant bone regions, while correctly classified normal cases show minimal activation. In contrast, misclassified samples tend to display scattered or misplaced attention, reflecting uncertainty in the model's decision-making.

4.3 Comparison with Prior Methods

Table 2. Comparison with Prior Methods

Method	VIS AUC	VIS F1 Score	INVIS AUC	INVIS F1 Score
ImageNet [20]	0.8961	80,00%	0.7549	72.70%
DRR20 [20]	0.9290	**85.20%**	0.8002	78.60%
ImageNet + DRR20 [20]	0.9280	83.90%	0.7140	72.10%
ImageNet + DRR20_Full [20]	0.9151	83.30%	0.6896	77.50%
PelFANet (Ours)	**0.9334**	84.71%	**0.8688**	**81.23%**

To validate the effectiveness of PelFANet, we compare it against multiple baselines from previous work that used ResNet-based classifiers [31] with various pretraining strategies, including ImageNet, Digitally Reconstructed Radiographs (DRR) synthetic data, and their combinations [21]. As shown in Table 2, PelFANet outperformed all prior models across both VIS and INVIS test sets.

On the VIS test set, PelFANet achieved an AUC of 0.9334, slightly outperforming the previous best method DRR20 with an AUC of 0.9290. More importantly, Despite being trained only on the VIS set, PelFANet showed a substantial improvement on the challenging INVIS subset, achieving an AUC of 0.8688 and an F1 score of 81.23%, which is significantly higher than the prior best DRR20 with an AUC of 0.8002 and F1 score of 78.60%.

This comparative analysis highlights the distinct advantage of our dual-input, attention-fused framework, which enables PelFANet to capture both global context from raw images and precise anatomical boundaries from segmentations. Unlike conventional single-stream or pretraining-only methods, our architecture dynamically refines features across both modalities through FABlocks and CBAM, leading to better performance especially when facing complex or subtle fracture patterns.

Despite the promising results, this work has several areas for further exploration. Our architecture combines segmentation with attention-based fusion to enhance fracture detection, but detailed ablations of components like CBAM and FABlocks are planned to better understand their impact. Pretraining on chest X-rays was chosen for their radiographic similarity and paired masks, though training from scratch will help assess the role of initialization. Comparisons were made using ResNet backbones to match prior work, and future evaluations will include modern architectures and other segmentation-guided or anatomy-aware approaches from related studies. Finally, we used bone segmentations over binary masks, assuming their richer detail aids classification, an aspect we plan to analyze further. These investigations will further strengthen the generalizability and interpretability of our approach.

5 Conclusion

In this study, we proposed PelFANet, a segmentation-guided dual-stream attention network designed to improve pelvic fracture classification, with a focus on invisible fractures. By integrating raw pelvic X-rays and corresponding bone segmentations, PelFANet leverages global anatomical context alongside localized structural cues. Its Fused Attention Blocks enable effective feature interaction between inputs, guiding the model to attend to diagnostically relevant regions. Results show PelFANet outperforms prior methods, especially in detecting invisible fractures, highlighting the potential of anatomy-aware dual-input models for real-world diagnostic challenges. However, further investigation is needed to fully understand the contributions of key components and to evaluate the model with more diverse architectures and datasets. Future work will address these limitations by expanding to other anatomical regions, incorporating more comprehensive ablations, and validating on larger, multi-center cohorts to support robust real-time clinical use.

Acknowledgments. We express our gratitude to Keigo Hayashi, Akihiro Maruo and Hirotsugu Muratsu from Hyogo Prefectural Harima-Himeji General Medical Center, Japan, for their valuable guidelines for data processing.

Disclosure of Interests. The Authors declare no competing interests.

References

1. Tile, M.: Pelvic ring fractures: should they be fixed? J. Bone Joint Surg. Br. **70**(1), 1–12 (1988)
2. Ferede, B., Ayenew, A., Belay, W.: Pelvic fractures and associated injuries in patients admitted to and treated at Emergency Department of Tibebe Ghion Specialized Hospital, Bahir Dar university, Ethiopia. Orthopedic research and reviews pp. 73–80 (2021)
3. Abdelrahman, H., et al.: Patterns, management, and outcomes of traumatic pelvic fracture: insights from a multicenter study. J. Orthop. Surg. Res. **15**(1), 249 (2020)

4. Ohla, J., et al.: Pelvic fractures in adults and the importance of associated injuries-a current multi-disciplinary approach. Clin. Pract. **15**(7), 130 (2025)
5. Weitz, M., Schwartz, C., Scheinfeld, M.H.: Radiologic blind spots in hip and pelvic radiographs. Emerg. Radiol. **30**(5), 569–575 (2023)
6. Pinto, A., et al.: Traumatic fractures in adults: missed diagnosis on plain radiographs in the emergency department. Acta. Bio. Medica. Atenei. Parmensis **89**(Suppl 1), 111 (2018)
7. Soto, J.R., Zhou, C., Hu, D., Arazoza, A.C., Dunn, E., Sladek, P.: Skip and save: utility of pelvic x-rays in the initial evaluation of blunt trauma patients. Am. J. Surg. **210**(6), 1076–1081 (2015)
8. Connor, G.S., McGwin Jr, G., Maclennan, P.A., Alonso, J.E., Rue III, L.W.: Early versus delayed fixation of pelvic ring fractures. Am. Surg. **69**(12), 1019–1024 (2003)
9. Kassem, M.A., Naguib, S.M., Hamza, H.M., Fouda, M.M., Saleh, M.K., Hosny, K.M.: Explainable transfer learning-based deep learning model for pelvis fracture detection. Int. J. Intell. Syst. **2023**(1), 3281998 (2023)
10. Tanzi, L., Vezzetti, E., Moreno, R., Aprato, A., Audisio, A., Massè, A.: Hierarchical fracture classification of proximal femur X-Ray images using a multistage Deep Learning approach. Eur. J. Radiol. **133**, 109373 (2020)
11. Luo, J., Sun, Y., Chi, J., Liao, X., Xu, C.: A novel deep learning-based method for covid-19 pneumonia detection from ct images. BMC Med. Inform. Decis. Mak. **22**(1), 284 (2022)
12. Ma, Y., et al.: Sg-transunet: A segmentation-guided transformer u-net model for kras gene mutation status identification in colorectal cancer. Comput. Biol. Medicine **173**, 108293 (2024)
13. Naaqvi, Z., Haider, M.A., Faheem, M.R., Ain, Q.U., Nawaz, A., Ullah, U.: Modified u-net model for segmentation and classification of liver cancer using ct images. J. Comput. Biomed. Inf. **6**(02), 1–12 (2024)
14. Zhou, Z., Rahman Siddiquee, M.M., Tajbakhsh, N., Liang, J.: UNet++: a nested U-Net architecture for medical image segmentation. In: Proceedings of DLMIA (2018)
15. Cao, H., et al.: Swin-Unet: Unet-like pure transformer for medical image segmentation. arXiv preprint arXiv:2105.05537 (2021)
16. Jaus, A., et al.: Anatomy-guided pathology segmentation. In: Linguraru, M.G., et al. (eds.) MICCAI 2024. LNCS, vol. 15008, pp. 3–13. Springer, Cham (2024). https://doi.org/10.1007/978-3-031-72111-3_1
17. Lee, J.M., Park, J.Y., Kim, Y.J., Kim, K.G.: Deep-learning-based pelvic automatic segmentation in pelvic fractures. Sci. Rep. **14**(1), 12258 (2024)
18. Lee, S.H., Jeon, J., Lee, G.J., Park, J.Y., Kim, Y.J., Kim, K.G.: Automated association for osteosynthesis foundation and orthopedic trauma association classification of pelvic fractures on pelvic radiographs using deep learning. Sci. Rep. **14**(1), 20548 (2024)
19. Cheng, C.-T., et al.: A scalable physician-level deep learning algorithm detects universal trauma on pelvic radiographs. Nat. Commun. **12**, 1066 (2021)
20. Chen, H., et al.: Anatomy-aware Siamese network: exploiting semantic asymmetry for accurate pelvic fracture detection in X-ray images. In: Vedaldi, A., Bischof, H., Brox, T., Frahm, J.-M. (eds.) ECCV 2020. LNCS, vol. 12368, pp. 239–255. Springer, Cham (2020). https://doi.org/10.1007/978-3-030-58592-1_15
21. Rahman, R., Yagi, N., Hayashi, K., Maruo, A., Muratsu, H., Kobashi, S.: Enhancing fracture diagnosis in pelvic X-rays by deep convolutional neural network with synthesized images from 3D-CT. Sci. Rep. **14**(1), 8004 (2024)
22. Woo, S., Park, J., Lee, J.Y., Kweon, I.S.: CBAM: convolutional block attention module. In: European Conference on Computer Vision (ECCV), pp. 3–19 (2018)
23. Ronneberger, O., Fischer, P., Brox, T.: U-net: convolutional networks for biomedical image segmentation. In: Navab, N., Hornegger, J., Wells, W.M., Frangi, A.F. (eds.) MICCAI 2015.

LNCS, vol. 9351, pp. 234–241. Springer, Cham (2015). https://doi.org/10.1007/978-3-319-24574-4_28
24. Xie, E., Wang, W., Yu, Z., Anandkumar, A., Alvarez, J.M., Luo, P.: SegFormer: simple and efficient design for semantic segmentation with transformers. Adv. Neural. Inf. Process. Syst. **34**, 12077–12090 (2021)
25. Tahir, A.M., et al.: COVID-19 infection localization and severity grading from chest X-ray images. Comput. Biol. Med. **139**, 105002 (2021)
26. Iakubovskii, P.: Segmentation Models Pytorch. GitHub repository. https://github.com/qubvel/segmentation_models.pytorch. Accessed 01 June 2025
27. Tahir, A.M., et al.: COVID-QU-Ex. Kaggle (2021)
28. Rahman, T., et al.: Exploring the effect of image enhancement techniques on COVID-19 detection using chest X-rays images. Comput. Biol. Med. 104319 (2021)
29. Degerli, A., et al.: Covid-19 infection map generation and detection from chest X-ray images. Health Inf. Sci. Syst. **9**, 15 (2021)
30. Chowdhury, M.E.H., et al.: Can AI help in screening viral and COVID-19 pneumonia? IEEE Access **8**, 132665–132676 (2020)
31. He, K., Zhang, X., Ren, S., Sun, J.: Deep residual learning for image recognition. In: IEEE Conference on Computer Vision and Pattern Recognition (CVPR), pp. 770–778 (2016)

XBoundNet++: Uncertainty-Aware Segmentation of Kidney Ablation Zones

Oren Arbel-Wood(✉), Maryam Rastegarpoor, and Aaron Fenster

Robarts Research Institute, Western University, London, Canada
{oarbelwo,mrasteg2,afenster}@uwo.ca

Abstract. Kidney ablation therapy is a minimally invasive procedure used to treat renal tumours. Evaluating treatment success for planning follow-up care relies on accurate kidney ablation zone (KAZ) segmentation in post-operative CT images. However, manual segmentation is time-consuming and prone to inter-observer variability and traditional segmentation is challenging as ground truth labels only provide a partial estimate of the area of interest. Segmenting the area of interest requires careful attention to the specific clinical needs of the resulting deep learning framework, including the addition of model interpretability and uncertainty estimation for further clinical review. We introduce a deep learning framework, XBoundNet++, that permits (1) precise segmentation of the boundary, (2) detailed attention maps for model layer-wise interpretability, and (3) model uncertainty estimation based on Bayesian Monte-Carlo dropouts and model ensembles. The model was trained and evaluated using a nested 5-fold cross-validation on a local dataset of 76 patients (with 912 CT 2D radial slices), collected at London Health Sciences Centre, which included manually annotated KAZs. Quantitative analysis showed that XBoundNet++ achieved promising segmentation results, including 88% precision, 83% recall, 84% DSC, 74% Jaccard, 6.89-pixel Mean Absolute Distance (MAD), -0.60-pixel Mean Signed Distance (MSD), and a 19.86-pixel Hausdorff distance (HD). Furthermore, heatmaps at each layer, probability and uncertainty maps, and uncertainty estimation at several thresholds indicate model trustworthiness, confidence, and justification for predictions. Our codebase can be found at https://github.com/oarbelw/XBoundNetPlusPlus and the dataset will be available upon request.

Keywords: Kidney Ablation · Segmentation · Interpretability · Uncertainty · Deep Learning · CT images

1 Introduction

Many segmentation methods perform well for known structures (e.g., kidney, liver in CT) [2, 17], as well as pathological structures (e.g., brain tumours) [18]. However, supervised learning requires the ground truth labels for objects of interest for training, but there are commonly contexts in which ground-truth labels are generally challenging to obtain. Furthermore, additional challenges are presented in these types of clinical contexts as they typically consist of a limited number of cases. These contexts are not well studied

N. Akash et al. (Eds.): EMERGE 2025 Workshops, LNCS 16534, pp. 114–123, 2026.
https://doi.org/10.1007/978-3-032-24182-5_11

in the literature and require particular care in terms of providing the clinician with model transparency and model uncertainty in order to trust the results and review the areas of relevance. This is crucial to enable trustworthy AI that aligns with established standards [14], helping with:

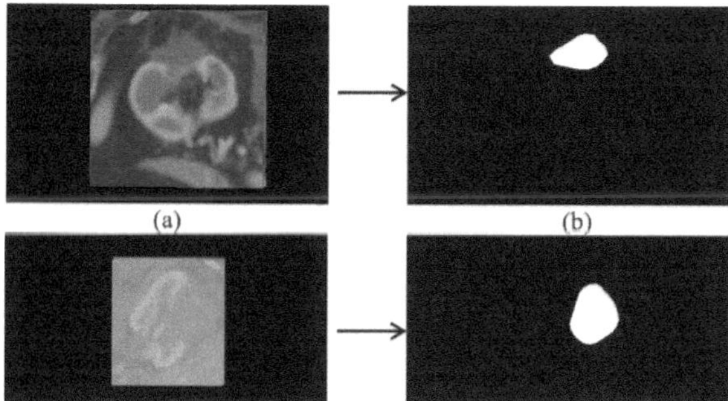

Fig. 1. Two sample patient images from the dataset, where (a) are raw images, and (b) clinically annotated images.

In this paper, we consider post-treatment delineation of the ablation zone in kidney CT images. Kidney cancer, or renal cell carcinoma, is one of the most prevalent urological malignancies worldwide. For patients unfit for surgical intervention, thermal ablation therapies like microwave or radiofrequency ablation offer a minimally invasive alternative. These procedures aim to destroy malignant cells by creating a "kidney ablation zone" (KAZ) that encapsulates the tumour and surrounding margin. Post-treatment assessment depends on accurately identifying the entirety of the KAZ in follow-up CT scans, which is a critical task for determining treatment success and guiding subsequent care [6].

The integration of uncertainty-aware deep learning techniques would be important in medical imaging domains involving ambiguous or low-contrast boundaries, such as post-ablation regions. However, to date, no deep learning models have been developed and published for this task.

Uncertainty estimation in deep learning models has been developed to help identify areas where predictions may be unreliable due to image ambiguity, label noise, or model uncertainty. A number of specific deep learning architectures were proposed to explicitly predict segmentation labels along with probabilistic outcomes, such as the Probabilistic U-Net [13] and PHISeg [1]. However, these models require architecture modification built specifically for particular kinds of uncertainty measures and are not easily adaptable to any context, for example, models that also embed attention modules within the framework. Other models were developed such as PULASki [3], a model that explicitly models inherent ambiguity arising from expert disagreement, and the recent Stochastic Segmentation Network (SSNs) [19], which specifically captures the aleatoric uncertainty seen in medical images.

In their seminal paper, Kendall and Gal [12] introduced a framework that models both aleatoric and epistemic uncertainty using Bayesian deep learning (BDL) techniques, which has become the foundation for uncertainty estimation in segmentation. BDL along with MC Dropout and deep ensembles permit a simple and effective mechanism for post hoc uncertainty estimates in several forms. The beauty of BDL models is that they can be used to estimate epistemic and aleatoric uncertainties through sampling techniques during inference for ANY network with dropout layers. As such, they are flexible and can be added to any network. They have been used in brain tumor segmentation [7, 15] and lesion segmentation [20]. In the context of kidney imaging, MC dropout has been used [25] in kidney tumors and cysts segmentation. While most segmentation studies [26] have focused on kidney tumors (e.g., the KiTS21 and KiTs23 datasets), segmentation of ablation zones, which present irregular, low contrast boundaries post-procedure, remains unexplored.

In this work, we introduce an *XBoundNet++*, an eXplainable Boundary-Aware modified ResU-Net++, a novel deep learning segmentation framework designed to provide clinicians with high-quality segmentation results, model transparency, interpretable tools, and uncertainty estimation using Bayesian Monte-Carlo (MC) dropout [8]. Our framework is aimed at shifting clinical practice from unclear binary masks to interpretable tools that explicitly provide confidence, uncertainty, probability, and transparency. We created an end-to-end pipeline to preprocess an image (as seen in Fig. 1), feed it into our model, generate segmentations of high quality that outperform other state-of-the-art models, provide comprehensive layer-wise transparency, and produce epistemic-uncertainty with probability maps.

2 Methods

2.1 XBoundNet++ Segmentation Network and Training

We propose XBoundNet++, an ensemble-based four-level modified U-Net [23] in Fig. 2, which introduces architectural elements that explicitly promote feature relevance, spatial focus, and post-hoc transparency. Our architecture integrates components from LeXNet++ [5], ResNet [9], attention mechanisms [21], Squeeze & Excitation (SE) [10], STEM [22], and several advanced architectures.

The Atrous Spatial Pooling Pyramid (ASPP) bridge, connecting the encoder and decoder, captured multi-scale context while maintaining dimensionality. It applied convolutions with dilations of 1, 6, 12, and 18 [4], performed a summation to merge the features, and applied a BN and ReLU activation.

Attention Gate blocks were introduced to selectively propagate relevant features during upsampling. They compute spatial attention maps via 1×1 convolutions and ReLU-sigmoid activation, suppressing irrelevant activations and enhancing decoder focus on the ablation zone.

The network was optimized with Adam (learning rate 10¯4, batch size 4) and a custom combined loss of Log-Dice ($\alpha = 0.7$) and binary cross-entropy ($\alpha = 0.3$), as Dice addresses class imbalance, while BCE improves per-pixel calibration, giving probabilistic outputs that can be further used for uncertainty estimation. Early stopping (patience = 50) and Reduce-LR-on-Plateau (factor 0.1, patience = 15) were employed to prevent over-fitting and facilitate convergence. The final combined loss is:

$$CombinedLoss(y, \hat{y}) = \alpha * LogDiceLoss(y, \hat{y}) + (1 - \alpha) * BCE(y, \hat{y}) \quad (1)$$

where y is the ground truth, ŷ is the prediction, and α is set to 0.7.

For each of the five patient-wise folds, we trained five instances of XBoundNet++ with differing seeds, yielding 25 independent models in total. Altering the seed affects weight initialization, alters the stochastic augmentation stream, and changes the sequence of dropout masks encountered during optimization. The resulting ensemble enhances predictive stability, generalizes the small dataset, and forms the basis for the uncertainty analysis described in the next section.

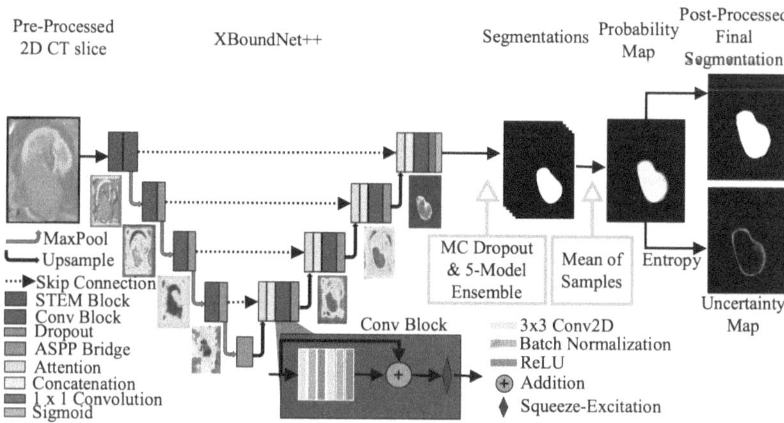

Fig. 2. Network pipeline and architecture with layer-wise activation maps.

2.2 Layer-Wise Heatmap Generation

We propose a custom Gradient-weighted Class Activation Mapping (Grad-CAM) [24] method that helps visualize which regions of an image had the most influence on the model by analyzing gradient-weighted activations that serve as spatial attention maps. First, the image is processed by the model, a class prediction is made, and during back-propagation, the gradients of the prediction are computed for the feature map at the chosen convolutional layer. Finally, the results are passed through a ReLU activation (and upsampled if necessary) to produce the heatmap for any given convolutional layer in the network.

We then extract heatmaps from every convolutional block across the network to observe how feature abstraction evolves at different depths. This strategy allows us to visually trace the information flow and decision-making within the network, revealing where and how the network's focus shifts, from low-level texture extraction to high-level semantic boundary recognition.

2.3 Model Inference and Uncertainty Estimation

During training, dropout mitigates over-fitting. During inference, the five seed-specific trained network models retained from each outer fold are evaluated with dropout kept active. For every unseen test slice, we generate 50 stochastic outputs using Bayesian MC dropout, yielding a collection of 250 predictions per slice. We then average this collection to create an ensemble-predictor, producing a probability map p for KAZ segmentation.

We use the probability map to generate an uncertainty map using normalized entropy, H, as a measure of uncertainty as portrayed below:

$$H = -[p\log(p) + (1 - p)\log(1 - p)]. \tag{2}$$

We pool the raw predictions of the validation slices and fit a one-dimensional logistic-regression calibrator. The fitted sigmoid is saved and applied to all test-set probabilities, producing a calibrated map. We then use a 0.4 threshold to binarize the prediction so that values are either 0 or 1. Next, we perform a morphological closing operation to seal small holes or gaps in the prediction if necessary. We also examined whether numerous disconnected components were present, in which case the largest foreground component is retained, and all other objects are suppressed. This didn't apply to instances where cysts are larger than the KAZ; in such a case, the second largest component is selected.

The cleaned final segmentation mask was then resized to the original CT image size (510×788 pixels) with Lanczos-4 interpolation and written to disk as an 8-bit BMP.

2.4 Evaluation Metrics

Standard pixel and distance-based metrics were used to assess both technical and clinical segmentation quality. These metrics included the Dice similarity coefficient (DSC), Precision, Recall, and Jaccard, which provide valuable quantitative insight on boundary overlap, precision, and quality of segmentation. Boundary accuracy was evaluated by the mean absolute distance (MAD), mean signed distance (MSD), and Hausdorff distance (HD), to quantify the comparative closeness and surface area.

To validate the segmentation uncertainty estimations, we apply thresholds. This involved normalizing the entropy estimates per slice ranged from 0 and 100, and varying the thresholds (T = 25, 50, 75) at different confidence levels as in [16]. Pixels exceeding the given threshold were labelled as uncertain and the remainder were cross-checked against the annotated mask to generate four disjoint classes: true positive (TP) (overlapping areas), false positive (FP) (over-prediction), false negative (FN) (under-prediction), and uncertain. As we lowered the uncertainty threshold, the FN and FP areas should have been filtered out while retaining the TP pixels. This validated that in areas where the model is confident, it is correct, while incorrect areas have high uncertainty. This permits clinical trust in areas of high model confidence. The entire spatial confidence map, along with the segmentation results, allows a framework for downstream clinical review.

3 Experiments and Results

3.1 Patient Data, Preprocessing and Implementation Details

Our patient dataset was collected after approval by the Western University Research Ethics Board using a GE Lightspeed 64-slice CT scanner and included 76 patients' cases, each containing 12 axial CT slices obtained post-ablation. All the images were in

DICOM format, grayscale, originally sized at 510 × 788 pixels, and were accompanied by manually annotated binary masks of the KAZ, which were generated by an expert. The 3D CT images were resliced radially around an approximate vertical axis of the KAZ every 15° into 2D CT images. This transformation ensured that the zone appears more consistently across 2D image samples. Each slice was resized to 256 × 256 pixels for computational feasibility to fit into the model, resulting in a dataset of 912 2D CT images, as shown in Fig. 1.

We normalized pixel intensities to a [0, 1] range, and split the dataset by patient into training (64%), validation (16%), and testing (20%) sets. This ensured that slices from the same patient did not appear in multiple subsets to avoid model bias. To enhance model reliability and reduce variance due to dataset partitioning, a nested 5-fold patient-wise cross-validation strategy was adopted. Each fold used a unique set of patients for training, validation, and testing, ensuring that no slices from a single patient were shared across splits.

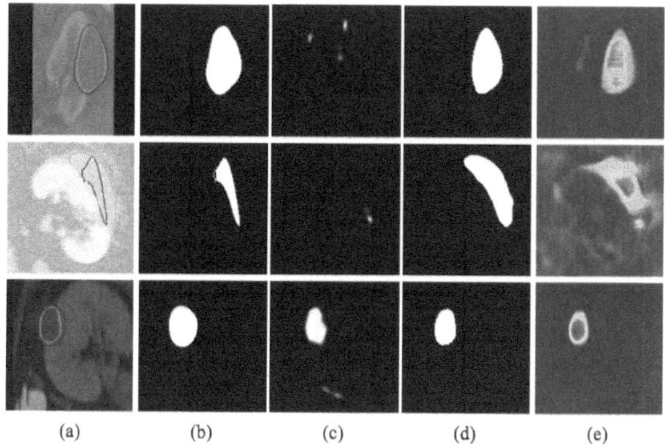

Fig. 3. XBoundNet++ results for three image slices from three different patients, in each row a) Original image, showing model prediction contour and clinical annotation, b) Clinically annotated mask, c) LeXNet++ prediction, d) XBoundNet++ prediction, e) The prediction attention heatmap from the convolutional layer before the sigmoid is applied. Attention shows higher gradient activation in red and thus more involvement in the resulting prediction, as it is more confident in the centre and is less confident at the boundaries.

On-the-fly data augmentation was applied to expand the appearance diversity while preserving label fidelity to compensate for the relatively small dataset. Augmentations were executed in TensorFlow eager mode, so a new stochastic version of every training image was generated for each epoch without materializing augmented files on disk. Each slice had a 30% chance of undergoing one or more spatial transformations: horizontal or vertical flip, translation of ±10% of the image extent, rotation of ±20°, or isotropic zoom between 0.9 and 1.1. Independently, there was a 30% chance of a photometric adjustment that scales contrast between 0.8 and 1.2.

3.2 Segmentation Results

Figure 3 shows the original image, mask, XBoundNet++ prediction, and the corresponding attention-based heatmap. These results show that the predictions generated by XBoundNet++ accurately align with the KAZ better than LeXNET++, as well as provide clarity on how strong the activations are that result in the arrival to the final prediction. This is evident in the first patient, where the KAZ, annotation mask, and model prediction all agree and cover the same area inside the kidney. While the second image may appear to be over-segmented, it is due to an incomplete annotation mask. The model correctly delineated the full ablation zone, outperforming the human annotation. The third prediction correctly under-segments, as the manual annotation extends beyond the actual KAZ and kidney region.

Table 1. Ablation analysis on different metrics in XBoundNet++, with the cumulative addition (+) of new components in descending order, highlighting the best result in grey.

Models \ Metrics	Precision	Recall	DSC	Jaccard	MAD (pixels)	MSD (pixels)	HD (pixels)
LeXNet++ Baseline	0.68±0.33	0.54±0.36	0.55±0.34	0.45±0.31	37.06±57.94	27.44±61.89	86.96±119.89
+XBoundNet++	0.71±0.20	0.68±0.30	0.66±0.27	0.54±0.26	26.00±41.83	17.59±44.03	61.95±66.28
+Augmentation	0.82±0.18	0.80±0.23	0.78±0.19	0.76±0.17	15.48±26.10	8.19±27.22	43.47±55.10
+Post-Processing	0.81±0.18	0.83±0.19	0.81±0.17	0.71±0.18	12.47±29.55	6.28±30.76	28.29±37.16
+CombinedLoss	0.84±0.18	0.82±0.19	0.82±0.17	0.72±0.17	10.54±24.13	3.80±25.39	24.83±31.64
+Ensemble	**0.88±0.11**	**0.83±0.13**	**0.84±0.10**	**0.74±0.13**	**6.89±4.33**	**-0.60±5.90**	**19.86±12.40**

The results of the ablation study are shown in Table 1 and were conducted to isolate the effect of each added XBoundNet++ component. Starting from the LeXNet++ [5] baseline, which lacks data augmentation, post-processing, and loss customization, we observe steady improvements across all metrics with each addition. XBoundNet++ alone improves DSC by 11%, recall by 14%, and HD by 25 pixels. Adding data augmentation further boosts DSC by 12%, Jaccard by 22%, and reduces MAD and MSD by over 9 pixels. Post-processing and the combined loss yield additional gains in boundary-related metrics, notably 3% DSC and a 15-pixel HD reduction. Finally, the ensemble improves all metrics, culminating in a 29% gain in DSC and Jaccard, 20% precision, and 67.1-pixel HD reduction compared to the baseline.

While these metrics demonstrate the quality of our proposed model, it is important to consider that there is no clear ground-truth in this application because KAZ boundaries are inherently ambiguous and the manually-drawn masks are subject to user variability. Thus, quantitative gains do not always capture the full clinical value (i.e., rows 2 and 3 in Fig. 3, where the model outperformed the annotation – based on post-hoc review).

3.3 Model Transparency

As visualized in Fig. 2, early convolutional layers tend to activate broadly across the ablation zone, while deeper layers increasingly emphasize peripheral boundary regions, particularly near ambiguous areas. The heatmaps clearly illustrate a transition from low-level texture detection in early layers to high-level semantic abstraction in deeper layers, confirming that the network progressively refines its attention toward clinically relevant boundaries. As a result, we can clearly track information flow and decision making, revealing the model's focus, enabling trustworthy AI.

3.4 Uncertainty Analysis

Figure 4 illustrates a qualitative analysis of a given patients' KAZ region and provides more insight for clinicians. The prediction doesn't span over the healthy tissue at the bottom despite the manual annotation including it. The clinician can refer to the probability and uncertainty overlays to manually scrutinize areas with less confidence and higher uncertainty. The results show that decreasing the threshold leads to filtering out pixels of high uncertainty only.

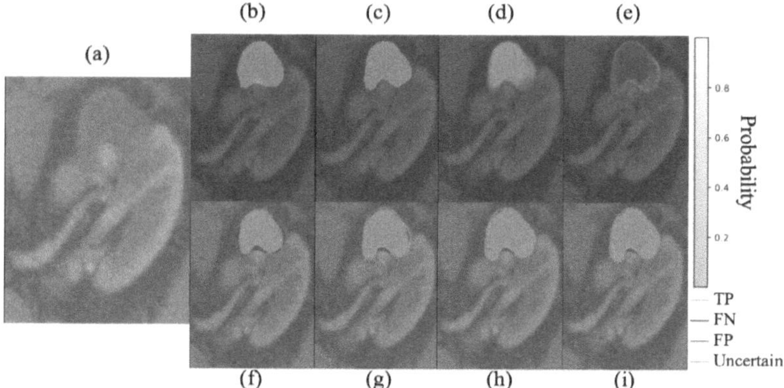

Fig. 4. XBoundNet++ results, uncertainty, probability, and thresholding visualized over a patient's CT slice. (a) CT original patient image slice, (b) Manually annotated mask, (c) XBoundNet++ predicted mask, (d) Probability map based on MC and ensembling, (e) Predicted entropy map from the probability map, (f) Uncertainty threshold = 100, (g) Uncertainty threshold = 75, (h) Uncertainty threshold = 50, (i) Uncertainty threshold = 25. It is desired that with more filtered out, more False Positives and False Negativespixels are filtered out (marked uncertain), while True Positivepixels remain unfiltered.

4 Conclusions

In this work, we propose XBoundNet++, a novel deep learning segmentation framework that provides clinicians with several auxiliary interpretable and uncertainty tools to better equip them for clinically challenging contexts such as poor image contrast, no delineated boundary, or incomplete labels. The model excels at segmentation based on several key metrics, provides in-depth transparency using Grad-CAM, and uncertainty estimation generated by Bayesian MC dropout and model ensembling. By offering transparency, spatial uncertainty, and probability overlays, XBoundNet++ enables more informed clinical review and supports safer, more trustworthy AI-assisted decision-making in interventional radiology.

The small dataset size, single-expert annotations, and use of 2D radial slices reflect common constraints in real-world clinical contexts. Rather than being limitations of the model, these challenges motivated our framework's design—tailored for clinically ambiguous labels and limited data. Standard models such as U-Net [23], while foundational in medical image segmentation, were not designed with uncertainty quantification or model transparency in mind. U-Net lacks mechanisms for epistemic or aleatoric uncertainty estimation, and offers no tools for layer-wise interpretability or confidence-guided clinical review—capabilities that are essential in interventional radiology. While adapting to 3D segmentation methods like nnU-Net [11] was not feasible in this setting as it requires large volumetric datasets and high-quality 3D annotations, future work will explore such extensions as larger, multi-center datasets and multi-rater annotations become available. We also aim to apply the model's uncertainty outputs to downstream tasks such as margin status, ablation volume, and residual tumour assessment.

Acknowledgments. The authors are grateful for funding from the Ontario Institute of Cancer Research (OICR) Grant RA#262 and the Canadian Institutes of Health Research (CIHR) – Grant FRN 154314.

Disclosure of Interests. The authors have no competing interests to declare that are relevant to the content of this article.

References

1. Baumgartner, C.F., et al.: PHISeg: capturing uncertainty in medical image segmentation. In: Shen, D., Liu, T., Peters, T.M., Staib, L.H., Essert, C., Zhou, S., Yap, P.-T., Khan, A. (eds.) MICCAI 2019. LNCS, vol. 11765, pp. 119–127. Springer, Cham (2019). https://doi.org/10.1007/978-3-030-32245-8_14
2. Çiçek, Ö., Abdulkadir, A., Lienkamp, S.S., Brox, T., Ronneberger, O.: 3D U-Net: learning dense volumetric segmentation from sparse annotation. In: Ourselin, S., Joskowicz, L., Sabuncu, M.R., Unal, G., Wells, W. (eds.) MICCAI 2016. LNCS, vol. 9901, pp. 424–432. Springer, Cham (2016). https://doi.org/10.1007/978-3-319-46723-8_49
3. Chatterjee, S., Honchar, A., Seibold, M., et al.: PULASki: learning inter-rater variability using statistical distances to improve probabilistic segmentation. Med. Image Anal. **85**, 103623 (2025)
4. Chen, L.-C., Papandreou, G., Kokkinos, I., Murphy, K., Yuille, A.L.: DeepLab: semantic image segmentation with deep convolutional nets, atrous convolution, and fully connected CRFs. IEEE Trans. Pattern Anal. Mach. Intell. **40**(4), 834–848 (2017)
5. Das, S., Khan, S.S., Sengupta, D., et al.: LeXNet++: layer-wise eXplainable ResUNet++ framework for segmentation of colorectal polyp cancer images. Neural Comput. Appl. (2024). https://doi.org/10.1007/s00521-024-10441-6
6. Escudier, B., Porta, C., Schmidinger, M., et al.: Renal cell carcinoma: ESMO clinical practice guidelines for diagnosis, treatment and follow-up. Ann. Oncol. **30**(5), 706–720 (2019)
7. Fuchs, M., Gonzalez, C., Mukhopadhyay, A.: Practical uncertainty quantification for brain tumor segmentation. In: Medical Imaging with Deep Learning (MIDL) (2021)
8. Gal, Y., Ghahramani, Z.: Dropout as a Bayesian approximation: representing model uncertainty in deep learning. In: ICML, pp. 1050–1059 (2016)
9. He, K., Zhang, X., Ren, S., Sun, J.: Deep residual learning for image recognition. In: IEEE Conference on Computer Vision and Pattern Recognition (CVPR), pp. 770–778 (2016)

10. Hu, J., Shen, L., Sun, G.: Squeeze-and-excitation networks. In: IEEE Conference on Computer Vision and Pattern Recognition (CVPR), pp. 7132–7141 (2018)
11. Isensee, F., Jaeger, P.F., Kohl, S.A.A., et al.: NnU-Net: a self-configuring method for deep learning-based biomedical image segmentation. Nat. Methods **18**, 203–211 (2021)
12. Kendall, A., Gal, Y.: What uncertainties do we need in Bayesian deep learning for computer vision? In: Advances in Neural Information Processing Systems (NeurIPS), vol. 20 (2017)
13. Kohl, S., Romera-Paredes, B., Meyer, C., et al.: A probabilistic U-Net for segmentation of ambiguous images. In: Advances in Neural Information Processing Systems (NeurIPS), vol. 31 (2018)
14. Lekadir, K., Frangi, A.F., Porras, A.R., Glocker, B., Cintas, C., Langlotz, C.P., et al.: FUTURE-AI: international consensus guideline for trustworthy and deployable artificial intelligence in healthcare. BMJ **388**, e081554 (2025)
15. Mehta, R., Paunovic, V., Arbel, T.: Propagating uncertainty across cascaded medical imaging tasks for improved deep learning inference. IEEE Trans. Med. Imaging **41**(11), 3090–3102 (2022)
16. Mehta, R.: Integrating Bayesian deep learning uncertainties in medical image analysis. Ph.D. thesis, Department of Electrical & Computer Engineering, McGill University (2023)
17. Meine, H., Chlebus, G., Ghafoorian, M., Endo, I., Schenk, A.: Comparison of U-net based convolutional neural networks for liver segmentation in CT. J. Intell. Fuzzy Syst. **83**, 71833–71862 (2024)
18. Menze, B.H., Jakab, A., Bauer, S., Kalpathy-Cramer, J., Farahani, K., Kirby, J., et al.: The multimodal brain tumor image segmentation benchmark (BRATS). IEEE Trans. Med. Imaging **34**(10), 1993–2024 (2015)
19. Monteiro, M., Allken, V., Wang, B., Jacob, M.W.: Stochastic segmentation networks: modelling spatially correlated aleatoric uncertainty. In: Advances in Neural Information Processing Systems (NeurIPS), vol. 33, pp. 12756–12767 (2020)
20. Nair, T., Chen, L., Yang, C., Precup, D.: Exploring uncertainty measures in deep networks for multiple sclerosis lesion detection and segmentation. Med. Image Anal. **59**, 101557 (2020)
21. Oktay, O., Schlemper, J., Le Folgoc, L., et al.: Attention U-Net: Learning where to look for the pancreas. arXiv preprint arXiv:1804.03999 (2018). https://arxiv.org/abs/1804.03999
22. Rastegarpoor, M., Cool, D.W., Fenster, A.: Segmentation of kidney ablation zone using deep learning in CT images. In: Proceedings of SPIE, vol. 13406, San Diego, USA (2025)
23. Ronneberger, O., Fischer, P., Brox, T.: U-Net: convolutional networks for biomedical image segmentation. In: Navab, N., Hornegger, J., Wells, W.M., Frangi, A.F. (eds.) MICCAI 2015. LNCS, vol. 9351, pp. 234–241. Springer, Cham (2015). https://doi.org/10.1007/978-3-319-24574-4_28
24. Selvaraju, R.R., Cogswell, M., Das, A., Vedantam, R., Parikh, D., Batra, D.: Grad-CAM: visual explanations from deep networks via gradient-based localization. Int. J. Comput. Vis. **128**(2), 336–359 (2019)
25. Salahuddin, Z., Zhang, T., Wang, Y., Salama, M.S.: Leveraging uncertainty estimation for segmentation of kidney, kidney tumor and kidney cysts. In: International Challenge on Kidney and Kidney Tumor Segmentation, pp. 40–46. Springer, Cham (2023). https://doi.org/10.1007/978-3-031-54806-2_6
26. Sudre, C.H., Dalca, A., Baumgartner, C.F.: Uncertainty for safe utilization of machine learning in medical imaging. In: MICCAI UNSURE Workshop (2022)

Self-supervised Vision Transformers for Prostate Cancer Classification in Biparametric MRI

Shebna Rose D. Fabilloren[1(✉)], Jose Conrado T. Paulino[2], Johanna Patricia A. Cañal[2], and Prospero C. Naval Jr.[1]

[1] University of the Philippines Diliman, Quezon City, Philippines
sdfabilloren@up.edu.ph

[2] University of the Philippines Manila, Manila, Philippines

Abstract. Multiparametric and biparametric magnetic resonance imaging (mpMRI/bpMRI) play an essential role in the detection, pre-biopsy planning, and staging of clinically significant prostate cancer (csPCA). One of the most commonly used structured reporting schemes in the evaluation of prostate MRI's for suspected prostate cancer is the Prostate Imaging–Reporting and Data System (PI-RADS) v.2.1, developed by multiple international representative groups. Existing machine learning models for classifying csPCa using PI-RADS are not reproducible due to the availability of data sets. Meanwhile, public datasets lack PI-RADS labels, a standard in prostate MRI. This hinders progress in the research community. FastMRI Prostate is a recently released, publicly available slice-level MRI dataset with PI-RADS labels. However, research using it is limited due to its recent release, and no studies have yet applied DINOv2 for csPCa classification on bpMRI. Several medical imaging studies have shown DINOv2 to be an effective feature extractor. This study aims to address these gaps by assessing the advantages and limitations of the DINOv2 family of foundation models on the FastMRI Prostate dataset for binary csPCa classification. Our findings reveal that DINOv2 models outperformed other ImageNet pretrained CNN-based models. ViT-g variant obtained an AUROC = 0.889 for the T2W model and 0.862 for the DWI model. This suggests DINOv2 features representations are adaptable to this downstream task. There was minimal performance difference between ViT-g and ViT-L, but a two-fold difference in training time and VRAM needed, making it a good alternative when computational resources are limited. ViT-S (21M parameters) achieved comparable performance to ResNet-152 (60M parameters). Overall, this suggests that DINOv2 models offer a good trade-off between performance and computational cost, making them a viable option even in resource-constrained environments.

Keywords: prostate cancer · vision transformer · biparametric mri

N. Akash et al. (Eds.): EMERGE 2025 Workshops, LNCS 16534, pp. 124–134, 2026.
https://doi.org/10.1007/978-3-032-24182-5_12

1 Introduction

Prostate cancer is a common health issue among the male population often present in men over 50 years old [4]. According to the Global cancer statistics (GLOBOCAN) in 2022, 1.5 million new cases of prostate cancer were registered worldwide [2]. This represents 7.3% of all cancers in men which made it rank second most common cancer. In terms of mortality, it is the fifth leading cause of cancer death in men worldwide. Male patients often seek medical consultation for lower urinary tract symptoms (LUTS), such as increased frequency, urgency, weak or intermittent stream, or difficulty emptying the bladder. Some present with more concerning signs like hematuria, anuria, or dysuria. Others may be asymptomatic but undergo prostate cancer screening based on age-specific clinical guidelines.

The first screening method for prostate cancer screening, after proper history taking and physical examination, is a digital rectal exam (DRE), where a medical professional inserts a finger into the rectum and palpates the prostate gland to provide a rough size measurement and to feel for irregularities in the prostate. However, many experts do not recommend this due to limited evidence of its benefits [11,15,22]. The second method is a blood test to measure prostate-specific antigen (PSA) levels. Elevated serum PSA levels may indicate prostate cancer, but may also show elevated results from non-cancerous conditions such as benign prostatic hyperplasia (BPH), which causes prostate enlargement, infections, or due to expected senescent changes, among other causes [13]. Patients with abnormal DRE or PSA results may then be referred for biopsy to confirm diagnosis, as a formal diagnosis of prostate cancer can only be done through histopathologic assessment after biopsy.

Transrectal ultrasound (TRUS)-guided prostate biopsy is a widely used diagnostic procedure for the detection of prostate cancer, typically performed in patients with elevated prostate-specific antigen (PSA) levels or abnormal digital rectal examination findings. Under real-time ultrasound guidance, tissue samples are systematically obtained–usually 10 to 12 cores–from different regions of the prostate for histopathologic evaluation. A pathologist then grades the samples using the Gleason scale [14]. As an invasive procedure, biopsy carries risks such as bleeding, pain, and infection. TRUS-guided biopsy also has a high false-negative rate due to blind sampling, as it often misses areas like the anterior gland, apex, and transition zone.

Pre-biopsy magnetic resonance imaging play an increasingly vital role in the early diagnosis of prostate cancer, and have been recommended prior to biopsies to avoid possible complications as well as false negative sampling. Multiparametric MRI (mpMRI) and biparametric MRI (bpMRI) are both used in prostate cancer imaging, each with distinct advantages and limitations. mpMRI combines T2-weighted (T2W), diffusion-weighted (DWI), and dynamic contrast-enhanced (DCE) imaging, offering high diagnostic accuracy, especially for clinically significant cancer. DCE improves lesion characterization in equivocal or small cases and is supported by clinical guidelines. However, mpMRI requires contrast administration, increasing scan time, cost, and risks in patients with renal insufficiency and may cause major adverse effects, including respiratory or cardiovascular issues and nephrogenic systemic fibrosis. In contrast, bpMRI omits DCE and relies only on T2W and DWI sequences. This approach significantly shortens the examination time, reduces costs, and eliminates the need for contrast, making it more accessible and safer for certain patient populations [10]. By using bpMRI, these issues are resolved while still producing similar results with mpMRI [3,5,16,23]. A limitation of bpMRI is its usage with the PI-RADS scoring system, specifically in the evaluation of the peripheral zone lesions with a DWI/ADC score of 3, which elevates to a score of 4 if significant contrast enhancement is detected. Prostate lesions detected on MRI can be graded using the Prostate Imaging–Reporting and Data System (PI-RADS) v2.1. This reporting system aims to standardize prostate MRI acquisition, interpretation, and reporting. The v2.1 scoring system ranges from 1 (very low likelihood of clinically significant prostate cancer, or csPCa) to 5 (very high likelihood). Scoring is based solely on MRI findings and excludes clinical history, digital rectal examination (DRE), and PSA levels.

Deep learning models require each input to have an expected outcome value, also known as a label, to learn the patterns behind the data. In terms of prostate MRI image PI-RADS scoring, the image dataset must contain enough samples for every PI-RADS score (i.e. 1 to 5) in order to learn the representation of each score. As highlighted in [1], it is important to have a benchmark dataset to ensure that research published can be beneficial to the public health community. Reproducible research by having a benchmark dataset is essential for advancing machine learning research in medical imaging.

Manual annotation of prostate MRI datasets is time and resource intensive, especially given the limited number of radiologists trained in this specialized type of imaging. The recently released FastMRI Prostate [21] dataset, which is publicly available, includes bpMRI scans with PI-RADS labels and slice-level annotations that reflect how radiologists assess the likelihood of clinically significant prostate cancer (csPCa). While the dataset has not yet been applied to prostate cancer classification tasks, its authors demonstrated feasibility of diagnosing csPCa by training a ConvNeXt [12] binary classification model on the provided slice-level labels. Huang et al. [9] showed that DINOv2 models performed best across three medical imaging benchmarks (i.e. Chest X-ray, iChallenge-AMD, HAM10000). This good performance indicates that features learned in the DINOv2 self-supervised training from a huge amount of data can be used for medical imaging. While DINOv2 has shown promise, its transferability to highly specialized modalities like MRI remains an open question. This makes it a viable option for testing vision foundation models on the FastMRI Prostate dataset. This research aims to address the lack of prior work done on binary csPCa classification using slice-level PI-RADS score labels on the prostate bpMRI. The primary contributions of our research are as follows:

- Application and limitations of DINOv2 on prostate MRI: We investigated all DINOv2 model sizes for the binary csPCa classification based on PI-RADS score labels and provide novel insights into its transferability, performance scaling, and domain-specific limitations in prostate MRI.

- Utilization of FastMRI Prostate dataset: We trained a classifier head on top of DINOv2 and CNN-based model backbones that can serve as future baseline performance on this novel dataset.

2 Methodology

2.1 Data

The FastMRI Prostate [21] dataset was used for linear probing various pretrained models such as DenseNet121 [8], ResNet152 [7], and VGG19 [20] pretrained on ImageNet1k [6], and DINOv2 [17] pretrained on a large, diverse, curated dataset of 142 million images via self-supervised learning. It contains T2W and DWI MRI sequences with PI-RADS labels indicating the existence and score of prostate cancer for each slice. In total, there are 312 subjects which are divided into training, validation, and test groups containing 218, 48, 46 subjects respectively. Table 1 shows the corresponding number of slices for each group including their distribution across PI-RADS categories (P = 1 to P = 5). For DWI, we only used the ADC map and b1500 DWI sequences.

Table 1. Distribution of MRI slices across data splits and PIRADS categories (abbreviated as P = 1 to P = 5) for T2W and DWI sequences.

MRI Seq.	Data Split	Total Slices	P = 1	P = 2	P = 3	P = 4	P = 5
T2W	Train	6,647	6,106	200	133	88	120
	Validation	1,462	1,345	23	67	10	17
	Test	1,399	1,290	41	31	10	27
DWI	Train	13,274	12,186	244	352	242	250
	Validation	2,916	2,672	38	142	18	46
	Test	2,790	2,578	46	78	56	32

2.2 Preprocessing

We trained two models for each MRI sequence. This is patterned after how clinicians use PI-RADS grading when assessing MRI sequences. Figure 2 shows a high-level flowchart of our training approach. In the T2W model, U-Net segmentation was applied to extract the region of interest (i.e. prostate area) in the T2W images [19]. U-Net has shown strong performance in prior studies involving segmentation in MRI data. Prostate segmentation was necessary because without it the model also takes into account the unrelated organs and tissues surrounding the prostate. This causes noise and affects the performance of the model. In addition, it aligns with the PI-RADS guidelines, which excludes the assessment of the peripheral zone in T2W images. The segmentation step resulted in a mask of the prostate region. The output image mask was cropped and resized to

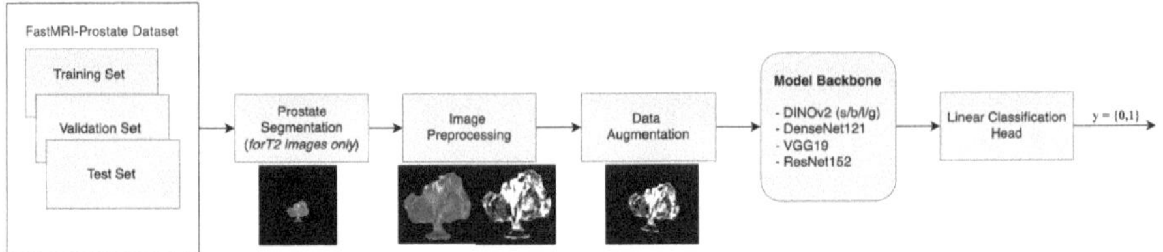

Fig. 1. End-to-end experiment pipeline. (a) Image preprocessing is composed of prostate segmentation (for T2W only), mask extraction, resizing, and normalization (b) Data augmentation involves translation, rotation, and horizontal flipping (c) The backbone weights are frozen (d) Linear classification head outputs 2 classes (0 = low risk, 1 = high risk)

224×224, then stacked to three channels to ensure compatibility with DINOv2's expected input shape. Data augmentation methods such as horizontal flipping, random rotation between -10 to $10°$, and translation, with limited minimum and maximum values for each axis, to avoid accidentally removing the region of interest in the augmented samples. Afterwards, normalization was applied to the images. The same preprocessing and augmentation steps were performed for the DWI model, except for prostate segmentation. ADC maps and b1500 DWI images were stacked after applying the preprocessing methods.

2.3 Training

All models were trained using PyTorch 2.0 [18] on NVIDIA RTX A6000 GPUs. The DINOv2 models were obtained from the official DINOv2 website. There are four backbones that vary according to the parameters they have. The classification head was left by default to show that linear probing is sufficient for the downstream task of csPCa classification. To avoid overfitting, several methods were performed. Cosine learning rate annealing was applied to stabilize model training. We used SGD optimizer with an initial value for learning rate set at $1e^{-5}$. Due to the nature of the problem where most samples will generally be non-csPCa, a weighted binary cross entropy loss function was applied to take into account the class imbalance.

$$\mathcal{L} = -\left(w_1 \cdot y \cdot \log(\hat{y}) + w_0 \cdot (1 - y) \cdot \log(1 - \hat{y})\right)$$

where $\mathcal{L}$ is the loss function:

- w_1 is the weight of the majority class
- w_0 is the weight of the minority class
- y is the true label
- $\hat{y}$ is the predicted label

The DenseNet121, VGGNet19, and ResNet152 models were obtained from the collection of readily available PyTorch models. These were already pretrained on the ImageNet [6] dataset. The model backbones were used as a feature extractor while a linear classification head was trained in the same manner as DINOv2 models to minimize the variation between the two groups. All of the models were trained with 20 epochs and a batch size of 32. The batch size was chosen as the maximum that can fit in the GPU resource used for this study. The only current model, as of writing, that has set an initial baseline performance for FastMRI Prostate dataset is the ConvNeXt architecture pretrained also on ImageNet. For each of these models, a linear classifier was trained on top of frozen pretrained features to evaluate downstream task performance. The end-to-end training pipeline is shown in Fig. 1.

Implementation code will be made available upon acceptance to ensure reproducibility.

3 Results and Discussion

3.1 Evaluation

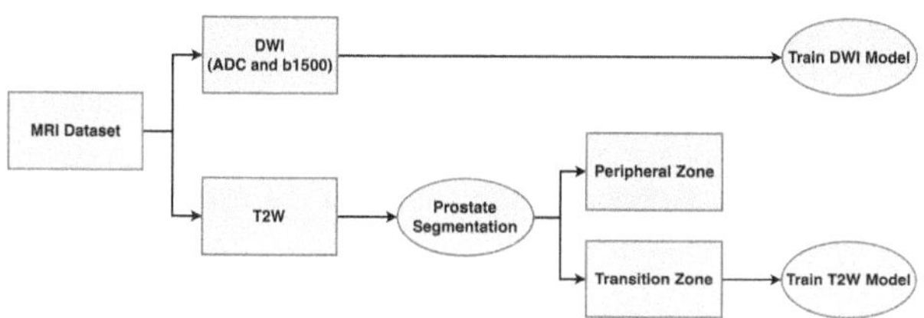

Fig. 2. Simplified flowchart on PI-RADS based on the MRI sequence.

Given the biparametric MRI input from FastMRI Prostate, two models were trained based on the zone of the prostate. This strategy was patterned after the PI-RADS assessment standards which suggests the use of T2W in assessing the transition zone and DWI for the peripheral zone. Each model will be able to focus on the characteristics of each MRI sequence. Final score is then evaluated in the same manner as clinicians do when referencing PI-RADS. Figure 2 shows the PI-RADS v2 assessment guidelines that clinicians use in assessing a prostate MRI.

Table 2. Comparison of AUC performance across all models

	DINOv2				CNN			
	ViT-S	ViT-B	ViT-L	ViT-g	ResNet-152	DenseNet-201	VGG-19	ConvNeXt
T2W	0.83	0.86	0.882	**0.889**	0.83	0.8	0.77	0.83
DWI	0.797	0.83	0.86	**0.862**	0.75	0.79	0.71	0.8

The model was evaluated using the area under the receiver operating characterstic curve (AUROC) in order to find out how well the model is able to classify. The task is approached as a binary classification problem, PI-RADS labels greater than or equal to 3 show high risk for csPCa requiring biopsy or other follow-up, and PI-RADS less than 3 indicates low risk for csPCa. This aligns with the clinically relevant threshold for distinguishing non-suspicious from suspicious findings. The developed model was tested against the test set of the FastMRI Prostate dataset and compared its performance against ImageNet pretrained CNN models.

3.2 Results

Table 2 shows that overall performance of DINOv2 pretrained models obtain a higher AUROC than the CNN-based models. An explanation for this is the quality of features learned by DINOv2 models during pretraining on a huge amount of unlabeled data, through self-supervised learning, compared to ImageNet1k. Specifically, the ViT-g variant obtained the highest score among all other methods for both the T2W model and DWI model. In comparison, the ViT-S variant scored similarly with other CNN-based models. Despite its significantly lower number of parameters (20M), it still achieves performance on par with ResNet152 (60M). It is expected that as the number of parameters increases, the performance also improves but only until a certain point. This can be observed with the score of ViT-L and ViT-g.

Table 3. Training (in minutes) and Inference Time (in milliseconds) for all DINOv2 model sizes including their corresponding number of parameters (in millions) and giga floating-point operations per second (GFLOPs) per image.

MRI Seq.	Variant	Params	GFLOPs	Training Time	Inference Time
T2W	ViT-S/14	20	≈ 4.5	1.77	0.78
	ViT-B/14	86	≈ 17	3.01	1.33
	ViT-L/14	300	≈ 61	6.02	2.66
	ViT-g/14	1,100	≈ 225	15.23	6.72
DWI	ViT-S/14	20	≈ 4.5	4.68	0.62
	ViT-B/14	86	≈ 17	9.5	1.28
	ViT-L/14	300	≈ 61	32.5	4.44
	ViT-g/14	1,100	≈ 225	118.2	16.21

Table 3 shows the wall-clock training and inference time for all DINOv2 models under the same hardware and software environment to ensure fair and consistent measurement. The time measurement includes the end-to-end pipeline from loading the image up to running the validation and test set evaluation. There

Table 4. Performance of the ViT-g model after individual preprocessing steps applied independently to T2W and DWI modalities. The baseline indicates performance without any preprocessing. Scores reflect AUC performance, and the absolute improvement compared to the baseline for each MRI sequence.

MRI Seq.	Preprocessing Step	AUC	Improvement
T2W	Baseline	0.720	–
	Center crop	0.833	0.113
	Zone segmentation + mask	0.865	0.145
	Horizontal flipping	0.840	0.120
	Rotation	0.840	0.120
	Translation	0.830	0.110
	Normalization	0.872	0.152
	All	**0.889**	**0.169**
DWI	Baseline	0.821	–
	Horizontal flipping	0.825	0.004
	Rotation	0.826	0.005
	Translation	0.830	0.009
	Normalization	0.847	0.026
	All	**0.862**	**0.041**

is minimal performance difference between the two models yet there is a two to four-fold difference in the training and inference time.

In Table 4, we show the effect of performing preprocessing on the model AUC scores. Ideally, DINOv2 features are ready to use for natural scene images. However, in the context of medical imaging, there is a domain shift that needs to be addressed. We explore if DINOv2 as a feature extractor on a linear classification head is capable of differentiating between csPCa and non-csPCa. For the T2W model, the baseline score is 0.72. Applying all preprocessing steps resulted in 0.169 increase which can be attributed to applying prostate zone segmentation (U-Net) and normalization. The T2W images need to be segmented as there are several organs visible in this MRI sequence. For this downstream task, we only need the prostate area, and referencing how clinicians use PI-RADS, the primary focus of T2W is for the transition zone only. Thus, it only makes sense to extract only the transition zone area of the prostate. In the DWI model, there is minimal improvement in the baseline (0.82) with just an increase of 0.041 after applying the preprocessing steps. Performing normalization contributed the most to the improvement as it standardizes the intensity distribution resulting in a better signal-to-noise ratio. This aligns with the PI-RADS as it focuses on the hypointensity for ADC and hyperintensity of high b-value DWI images. Despite adding a few preprocessing steps, this does not significantly affect the time it takes to train the model or perform inference.

3.3 Limitations and Future Work

This study utilized minimal preprocessing and a simple classification head to evaluate the capabilities of feature extractors, particularly DINOv2's backbones, without extensive customization. The scope was limited to binary classification to establish the potential of DINOv2 for prostate cancer detection on bpMRI. Additionally, while this study focuses on linear probing, fine-tuning offers a promising avenue for future improvement. Future work will expand to multi-class classification using the full PI-RADS scoring system (1–5). While the T2W model showed promising results, its performance may improve with advanced prostate segmentation techniques. Beyond the benchmark dataset, we are now evaluating the method on clinical MRI data from a tertiary hospital to assess the method's performance in real-world settings and its potential for clinical use.

4 Conclusion

This study highlights the advantages and limitations of DINOv2 in 2D binary classification when applied to FastMRI Prostate. The ViT-g variant obtained the highest AUROC for both T2W and DWI models. Despite freezing the backbone which allowed it to act as a feature extractor, it still achieved strong performance. However, training required significant VRAM ($\approx$ 46 GB). Given minimal performance differences, the ViT-L variant is a more resource-efficient alternative, using roughly half the VRAM of ViT-g. A key strength of the DINOv2 models lies in the high-quality feature representations learned during large-scale pretraining. Future work will extend to 2D multi-class classification across all PI-RADS classes using the FastMRI Prostate dataset.

Acknowledgement. This study was funded by the University of the Philippines Intelligent Systems Center (ISRGA2024-24).

Disclosure of Interests. The authors have no competing interests to declare that are relevant to the content of this article.

References

1. Bell, L.C., Shimron, E.: Sharing data is essential for the future of AI in medical imaging. Radiol. Artif. Intell. **6**(1), e230337 (2024). https://doi.org/10.1148/ryai.230337
2. Bray, F., et al.: Global cancer statistics 2022: GLOBOCAN estimates of incidence and mortality worldwide for 36 cancers in 185 countries. CA Cancer J. Clin. **74**(3), 229–263 (2024). https://doi.org/10.3322/caac.21834
3. Brembilla, G., et al.: Diagnostic accuracy of abbreviated bi-parametric MRI (a-bpMRI) for prostate cancer detection and screening: a multi-reader study. Diagnostics **12**(2), 231 (2022). https://doi.org/10.3390/diagnostics12020231
4. Centers for Disease Control and Prevention: Basic Information About Prostate Cancer (2022). https://www.cdc.gov/cancer/prostate/basic_info/index.htm

5. Choi, M.H., Kim, C.K., Lee, Y.J., Jung, S.E.: Prebiopsy biparametric MRI for clinically significant prostate cancer detection with PI-RADS version 2: a multicenter study. Am. J. Roentgenol. **212**(4), 839–846 (2019). https://doi.org/10.2214/AJR.18.20498
6. Deng, J., Dong, W., Socher, R., Li, L.J., Li, K., Fei-Fei, L.: Imagenet: a large-scale hierarchical image database. In: 2009 IEEE Conference on Computer Vision and Pattern Recognition, pp. 248–255 (2009). https://doi.org/10.1109/CVPR.2009.5206848
7. He, K., Zhang, X., Ren, S., Sun, J.: Deep residual learning for image recognition. In: 2016 IEEE Conference on Computer Vision and Pattern Recognition (CVPR), pp. 770–778. IEEE, Las Vegas, NV, USA (2016). https://doi.org/10.1109/CVPR.2016.90
8. Huang, G., Liu, Z., Van Der Maaten, L., Weinberger, K.Q.: Densely connected convolutional networks. In: 2017 IEEE Conference on Computer Vision and Pattern Recognition (CVPR), pp. 2261–2269. IEEE, Honolulu, HI (2017). https://doi.org/10.1109/CVPR.2017.243
9. Huang, Y., et al.: Comparative analysis of ImageNet pre-trained deep learning models and DINOv2 in medical imaging classification. In: 2024 IEEE 48th Annual Computers, Software, and Applications Conference (COMPSAC), pp. 297–305. IEEE Computer Society, Los Alamitos, CA, USA (2024). https://doi.org/10.1109/COMPSAC61105.2024.00049
10. Ibrahim, M.A., Hazhirkarzar, B., Dublin, A.B.: Gadolinium magnetic resonance imaging. In: StatPearls. StatPearls Publishing, Treasure Island (FL) (2025). http://www.ncbi.nlm.nih.gov/books/NBK482487/
11. Krilaviciute, A., et al.: Digital rectal examination is not a useful screening test for prostate cancer. Eur. Urol. Oncol. **6**(6), 566–573 (2023). https://doi.org/10.1016/j.euo.2023.09.008
12. Liu, Z., Mao, H., Wu, C.Y., Feichtenhofer, C., Darrell, T., Xie, S.: A convnet for the 2020s. In: Proceedings of the IEEE/CVF Conference on Computer Vision and Pattern Recognition (CVPR) (2022)
13. McNally, C.J., Ruddock, M.W., Moore, T., McKenna, D.J.: Biomarkers that differentiate benign prostatic hyperplasia from prostate cancer: a literature review. Cancer Manag. Res. **12**, 5225–5241 (2020). https://doi.org/10.2147/CMAR.S250829
14. Moe, A., Hayne, D.: Transrectal ultrasound biopsy of the prostate: does it still have a role in prostate cancer diagnosis? Transl. Androl. Urol. **9**(6), 3018–3024 (2020). https://doi.org/10.21037/tau.2019.09.37
15. Naji, L., et al.: Digital rectal examination for prostate cancer screening in primary care: a systematic review and meta-analysis. Ann. Family Med. **16**(2), 149–154 (2018). https://doi.org/10.1370/afm.2205
16. Noh, T.I., et al.: Comparison between biparametric and multiparametric MRI in predicting muscle invasion by bladder cancer based on the VI-RADS. Sci. Rep. **12**(1), 20689 (2022). https://doi.org/10.1038/s41598-022-19273-7
17. Oquab, M., et al.: Dinov2: learning robust visual features without supervision (2023)
18. Paszke, A., et al.: PyTorch: An Imperative Style, High-performance Deep Learning Library. Curran Associates Inc., Red Hook (2019)
19. Ronneberger, O., Fischer, P., Brox, T.: U-Net: convolutional networks for biomedical image segmentation. In: Navab, N., Hornegger, J., Wells, W.M., Frangi, A.F. (eds.) MICCAI 2015. LNCS, vol. 9351, pp. 234–241. Springer, Cham (2015). https://doi.org/10.1007/978-3-319-24574-4_28

20. Simonyan, K., Zisserman, A.: Very deep convolutional networks for large-scale image recognition. In: International Conference on Learning Representations (2015)
21. Tibrewala, R., et al.: FastMRI Prostate: a public, biparametric MRI dataset to advance machine learning for prostate cancer imaging. Sci. Data **11**(1), 404 (2024). https://doi.org/10.1038/s41597-024-03252-w
22. US Preventive Services Task Force, et al.: Screening for prostate cancer: US preventive services task force recommendation statement. JAMA **319**(18), 1901 (2018). https://doi.org/10.1001/jama.2018.3710
23. Xu, L., et al.: Comparison of biparametric and multiparametric MRI in the diagnosis of prostate cancer. Cancer Imaging **19**(1), 90 (2019). https://doi.org/10.1186/s40644-019-0274-9

Memory-Enhanced Temporal Learning: Leveraging SAM2's Memory Modules for Consistent Segmentation on Surgical Video

Shunsuke Kikuchi[1,2](✉), Atsushi Kouno[1], and Hiroki Matsuzaki[1]

[1] Jmees Inc., Kashiwa, Chiba, Japan
shunkikuchi2111@ucla.edu
[2] Computational and Systems Biology Program, UCLA, Los Angeles, CA 90095, USA

Abstract. Video segmentation is critical for many medical imaging applications; however, developing video-aware models is challenging as they require densely annotated large-scale datasets. Most mainstream segmentation models process each frame independently, often resulting in inconsistent segmentation masks across consecutive frames. Although the recently proposed Segment Anything Model 2 (SAM2) has demonstrated promising segmentation capabilities with its memory mechanism, applying SAM2 in clinical settings is challenging due to its reliance on user prompts.

To address these issues, we introduce the Temporal Memory Augmentation Module (TMAM). TMAM adapts any pre-trained 2D segmentation model by encoding past-frame predictions via SAM2's memory encoder and applying memory attention to refine current-frame features. By leveraging temporal redundancy in video sequences, TMAM captures contextual cues that may be overlooked by single-frame processing, thereby improving robustness to occlusions and boundary artifacts.

Experiments on public surgical video datasets demonstrate that TMAM enhances Dice scores and temporal consistency across various base architectures. These results highlight TMAM's ability to produce smoother, more coherent segmentations, paving the way for more reliable video analysis in surgical image navigation systems and robotic surgery, where precise and consistent segmentation is essential.

Keywords: Video Segmentation · Endoscopic Video · Temporal Consistency

1 Introduction

Accurate and temporally consistent video segmentation is crucial in medical image analysis, particularly for high-stakes applications such as surgical support systems and robotic surgery. In these settings, reliable segmentation not only

N. Akash et al. (Eds.): EMERGE 2025 Workshops, LNCS 16534, pp. 135–144, 2026.
https://doi.org/10.1007/978-3-032-24182-5_13

enhances the precision of tissue and instrument tracking but also directly contributes to improved patient outcomes. Recent advances, exemplified by the Segment Anything Model 2 (SAM2), have demonstrated that incorporating memory mechanisms to capture temporal context can dramatically enhance segmentation performance [11].

Based on recent trends in MICCAI EndoVis Challenges [10,13,18], the main approach for organ and instrument segmentation has been to apply frame-by-frame segmentation models to videos. This method tends to yield stable performance, particularly in challenging and data-scarce medical imaging scenarios. However, this approach fails to leverage the rich temporal continuity inherent in video data—an issue that is particularly pronounced in medical videos, where occlusions, rapid motion, and partial object appearances are common, and temporally dense annotations are rarely available.

On the other hand, video-specific segmentation methods have been proposed [2,5,8]. Yet, adapting such models to the medical domain is nontrivial; high training costs, the need for temporally dense annotations, and prolonged training times pose significant challenges. Moreover, while considerable progress has been made in video segmentation for natural images, methods tailored for medical videos—characterized by subtle anatomical differences and limited data—remain sparse.

Motivated by these challenges, we propose the **Temporal Memory Augmentation Module (TMAM)**. By leveraging transfer learning, TMAM reduces the cost of learning temporal information and effectively extracts and integrates temporal redundancy from even sparsely annotated medical video datasets. TMAM transfers SAM2's memory encoder and memory attention mechanisms to enhance existing 2D segmentation architectures. The key contributions of our paper are:

1. By integrating past-frame predictions through a memory encoder and refining current-frame features via memory attention, our approach mitigates inconsistencies caused by occlusions and boundary artifacts while significantly improving temporal coherence. It is expected to provide stable boundaries in long surgical videos, resulting in easily interpretable masks for humans and noise free for the surgical system.
2. The TMAM is designed as a plug-and-play module compatible with all encoder-decoder segmentation architectures, seamlessly enabling temporal inference capabilities without extensive modifications.
3. The TMAM leverage a domain-specific encoder during the frame propagation process, which is not possible with the standard SAM2 framework. This allows TMAM to recover from initial prediction errors and robustly handle challenges like occlusions
4. Furthermore, regarding automation, a simple tracking approach based on SAM2 would fail as the video progresses. It cannot predict instruments or organs that appear after the initial frame. Requiring new prompts for every new object during a surgical procedure is impractical. TMAM solves this by enabling true end-to-end automatic segmentation.

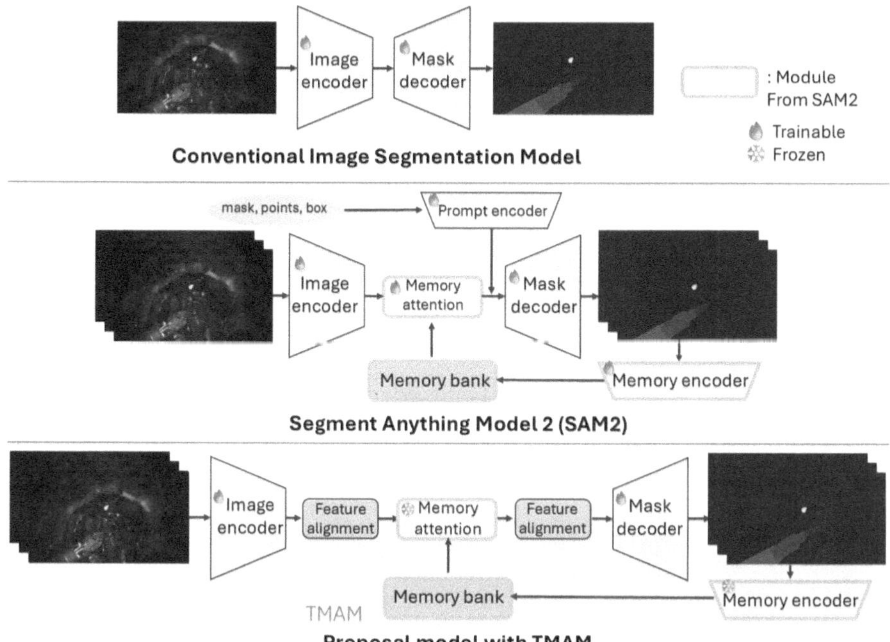

Fig. 1. Comparison of Conventional segmentation model, SAM2, and our proposed model incorporates a Temporal Memory Alignment Module (TMAM) to enhance feature consistency and segmentation accuracy. Trainable and frozen components are indicated.

2 Methods

Overall Framework. Figure 1 illustrates the architecture of TMAM and its functionality. TMAM is designed to integrate with any pretrained 2D segmentation model consisting of an encoder and decoder. It incorporates the memory encoder and memory attention components from SAM2.1-base, performing feature alignment to adjust tensor sizes and dimensions. With this alignment, TMAM performs segmentation without the prompts required in SAM2. Additionally, TMAM employs an internal memory module that stores temporal representations from previous frames, which are retrieved during memory attention to refine current-frame predictions.

Memory Attention. The deepest feature map from the encoder is resized to 64 × 64, then reshaped to match the channel dimensions required by the memory-attention mechanism. Following the cross-attention operation, the refined feature map is resized back to its original resolution and passed to the decoder. The mask for the first frame is generated using the base model, skipping the memory attention module. To ensure consistency, we reuse SAM2's positional encoding.

Feature Alignment, Memory Encoder and Module. For multi-class segmentation, a single-channel mask is generated by inverting the background probability. The memory encoder produces a 64×64 tensor, reshaped to (B,H×W,C). At each new frame, memory representations from the 10 most recent frames are concatenated along the batch dimension. This aggregated memory is stored internally and utilized by the memory-attention mechanism to integrate contextual information from prior frames.

3 Experiments

3.1 Experimental Setup

SAR-RARP50. This is a publicly available dataset. We adopt the data split as described in the original SAR-RARP50 paper [10]. This dataset contains surgical videos with nine instrument classes, annotated every 60 frames.

CholecSeg8k. This is a dataset consists of 8,080 pixel-wise annotated frames extracted from 17 laparoscopic cholecystectomy videos in the Cholec80 dataset. Each frame includes semantic segmentation masks for 13 anatomically and surgically relevant classes, supporting detailed analysis of endoscopic scenes. [4]

Training Settings. We first trained baseline models (e.g., U-Net [12]/EfficientNet-B7 [15], U-Net/MaxViT-T [16], DeepLabV3+ [1]/ResNet-101 with RAdamSchedulefree [3]. The learning rate is set to 1×10^{-4} for MaxViT encoders and 1×10^{-3} otherwise. The models were trained for 75 epochs with a batch size of 16, applying TrivialAugment [9]. For TMAM fine-tuning and ablation studies, no augmentation was applied. We used a batch size of 1 and trained for three epochs, including unlabeled frames to facilitate learning of temporal relationships. Both training and fine-tuning utilized Generalized Dice Focal Loss, defined as:

$$\mathcal{L}_{\text{total}} = \mathcal{L}_{\text{GeneralizedDice}} + \mathcal{L}_{\text{Focal}} \tag{1}$$

where $\mathcal{L}_{\text{GeneralizedDice}}$ is Generalized Dice Loss [14], and $\mathcal{L}_{\text{Focal}}$ is Focal Loss [6].

Evaluation Metrics. We measure spatial segmentation accuracy using the per-class Dice Score, calculated for each individual image and then averaged. To assess temporal consistency, we modified the approach defined in [7]. Instead of using the original implementation, we employed RAFT [17] to predict optical flow between consecutive frames. The mask $t-1$ is warped to frame t using the predicted flow, and the mean Intersection over Union (mIoU) is computed between the warped mask and the predicted mask for frame t. This metric is averaged across all frames in each video. For each dataset, temporal consistency is evaluated at fps = 60 (SAR-RARP50) and fps = 25 (CholecSeg8k).

Ablation Study. An ablation study was conducted to isolate the effect of TMAM. Using the same training settings—minimal augmentation with resizing only, batch size 1, and 3 epochs, we fine-tuned the base segmentation models both with and without the TMAM components.

Implementation Details. All experiments were conducted on a system equipped with an NVIDIA Quadro RTX 8000 GPU (48 GB VRAM) running Ubuntu 22.04.3 LTS. The CPU is an AMD EPYC 7702P 64-Core Processor. The source Code is available at: https://github.com/JmeesInc/TMAM.

3.2 Results

Table 1. SAR-RARP50: Average Dice and average Temporal Consistency (TC) at 60 fps. * means additional training on 3 epochs for ablation study. Proposal method is indicated by (+TMAM).

Model	Dice	TC@60fps
DeepLabV3+/ResNet-101	0.913	0.662
DeepLabV3+/ResNet-101*	0.907	0.657
DeepLabV3+/ResNet-101(+**TMAM**)	**0.922**	**0.673**
U-Net/EfficientNet-B7	0.867	0.608
U-Net/EfficientNet-B7*	0.865	0.604
U-Net/EfficientNet-B7(+**TMAM**)	**0.877**	**0.654**
U-Net/MaxViT-T	0.872	0.583
U-Net/MaxViT-T*	0.882	0.590
U-Net/MaxViT-T(+**TMAM**)	**0.923**	**0.669**

Table 2. CholecSeg8k: Average Dice and average Temporal Consistency (TC) at 25 fps. * means additional training on 3 epochs for ablation study. Proposal method is indicated by (+TMAM).

Model	Dice	TC@25fps
DeepLabV3+/ResNet-101	0.844	0.645
DeepLabV3+/ResNet-101*	0.842	0.645
DeepLabV3+/ResNet-101(+**TMAM**)	**0.873**	**0.686**
U-Net/EfficientNet-B7	0.869	0.608
U-Net/EfficientNet-B7*	0.872	0.609
U-Net/EfficientNet-B7(+**TMAM**)	**0.877**	**0.647**
U-Net/MaxViT-T	0.867	0.574
U-Net/MaxViT-T*	0.866	0.572
U-Net/MaxViT-T(+**TMAM**)	**0.872**	**0.577**

Table 1 summarizes the experimental results for the SAR-RARP50 dataset across three base model configurations. In each configuration, incorporating TMAM improves the Dice Score by approximately 1 to 4% points on average compared to the corresponding 2D model. TMAM also consistently enhances temporal consistency, yielding an improvement of around 15% points for the first two models equipped with U-Net. Notably, temporal consistency improvements are observed.

Table 2 shows the results for the CholecSeg8k dataset. While the Dice Score improvements with TMAM are more limited depending on the model, TMAM consistently leads to performance gains across configurations.

The inference speed was not significantly different from SAM2, ran at 4 FPS on our system. The slowest configuration (ResNet+DeepLabV3+) ran at 2 FPS, while the fastest (MaxViT-UNet++) achieved 9 FPS.

3.3 Qualitative Evaluation

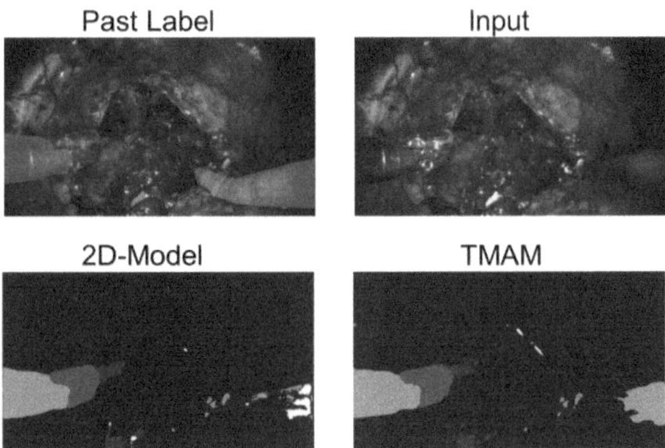

Fig. 2. Comparison under extreme motion. TMAM leverages temporal context to accurately segment the heavily blurred input frame (upper right). The ground truth (upper left) is from a previous, clearer frame. Sample: Video 11-1, index 180 (GT) & 210 (input).

In addition to quantitative metrics, we conducted a qualitative analysis in challenging scenarios. First, we examine cases where single-frame information is severely compromised. In Fig. 2, extreme motion blur significantly degrades the input image. In Fig. 3, the input image has extreme dark regions. In both cases, while 2D model fails to capture the accurate contour and instance classes, TMAM successfully reconstructs the scene and delivers a precise segmentation.

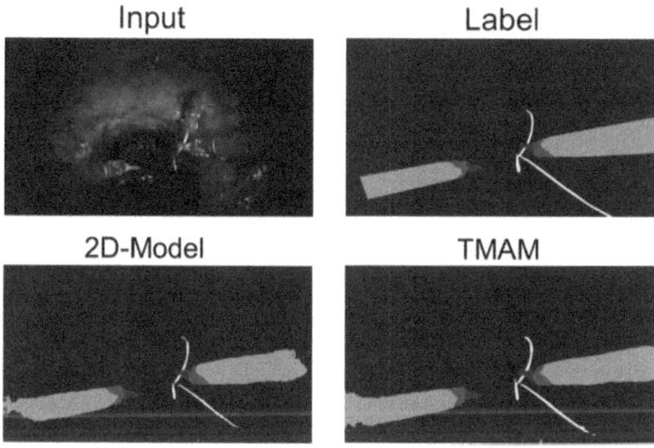

Fig. 3. Comparison in a low-light scenario. TMAM accurately segments the instrument in the dark, where the baseline model fails. Sample: Video 2, index 960.

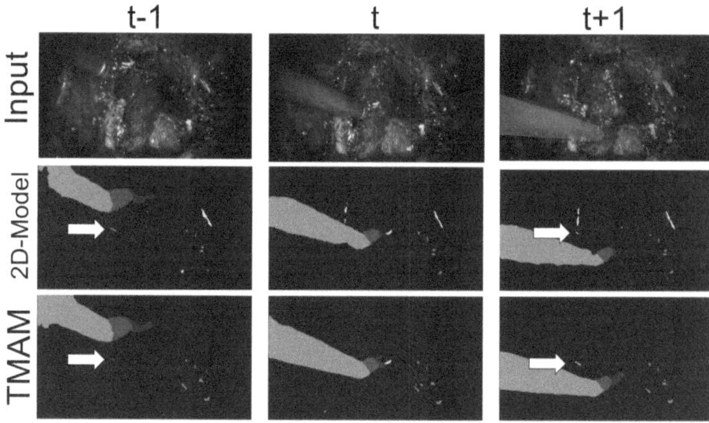

Fig. 4. Temporal consistency during an occlusion. The white arrow indicates the instrument hidden at frame t. TMAM retains the object's memory, ensuring consistent segmentation at frame $t + 1$. Sample: Video 36, indices 120, 180, 240.

Next, we evaluate the crucial aspect of temporal consistency, especially during events like occlusion and partial visibility. Figure 4 illustrates an occlusion scenario where an instrument is temporarily hidden. While 2D models lose track of such objects, TMAM retains the instrument class once it reappears. Figure 5 further demonstrates this capability in a scenario with limited visibility, where TMAM correctly identifies an instrument whose key features are off-camera by recalling its appearance from memory.

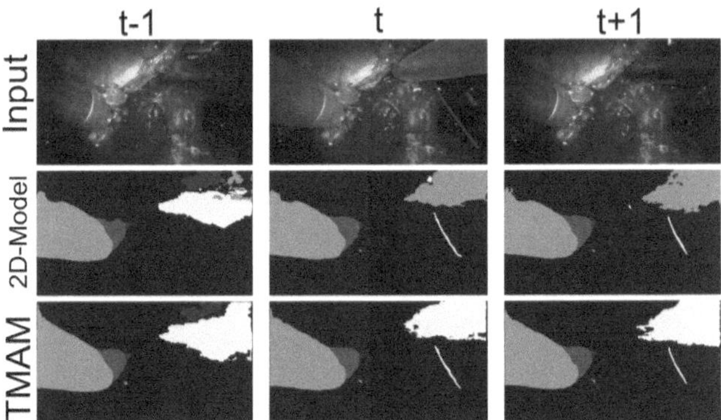

Fig. 5. Temporal consistency with limited visibility. TMAM correctly identifies the partially visible instrument at frame t by recalling its appearance from memory. Sample: Video 7, indices 1500, 1560, 1620.

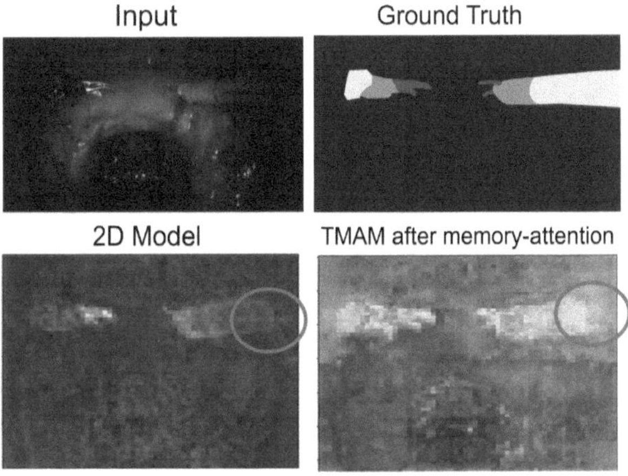

Fig. 6. Comparison of feature map between 2D model and TMAM.

4 Discussion and Conclusion

Analysis of the feature maps in Fig. 6 further demonstrates that the memory-attention mechanism compensates for critical temporal features often overlooked by single-frame models. Comparing the input image, feature maps from a conventional 2D model, and those before and after TMAM's memory-attention suggests that TMAM enriches feature representations by integrating information from past frames.

Despite these promising results, the computational cost of TMAM remains high. Future work should explore strategies to reduce this complexity. Ensuring real-time capability is crucial for clinical applications; therefore, optimizing the inference pipeline to minimize latency while maintaining accuracy is a critical direction for further research.

In conclusion, our study demonstrates that TMAM significantly enhances both spatial segmentation accuracy and temporal consistency across different base models and datasets. These improvements are particularly pronounced in multi-class surgical tool segmentation, where zero-shot methods fall short, and in high-difficulty tasks. These advancements pave the way for more reliable and robust segmentation systems in medical video analysis, ultimately contributing to enhanced surgical precision and patient safety.

Supplementary Material. A video used for validation with, TMAM inference, base model inference, and ground truth is available from github repository.

Disclosure of Interests. Shunsuke Kikuchi received financial support for a research internship at Jmees Inc. Atsushi Kouno is an employee of Jmees Inc. Hiroki Matsuzaki is the co-founder and CEO of Jmees Inc.

References

1. Chen, L.C., Zhu, Y., Papandreou, G., Schroff, F., Adam, H.: Encoder-decoder with atrous separable convolution for semantic image segmentation. In: ECCV (2018)
2. Cheng, H.K., Oh, S.W., Price, B., et al.: Putting the object back into video object segmentation. In: Proceedings of the IEEE/CVF Conference on Computer Vision and Pattern Recognition (CVPR), pp. 3151–3161 (2024)
3. Defazio, A., Yang, X., Mehta, H., et al.: The road less scheduled (2024)
4. Hong, W.Y., Kao, C.L., Kuo, Y.H., Wang, J.R., Chang, W.L., Shih, C.S.: Cholecseg8k: a semantic segmentation dataset for laparoscopic cholecystectomy based on cholec80 (2020). https://arxiv.org/abs/2012.12453
5. Li, X., Zhang, W., Pang, J., et al.: Video k-net: a simple, strong, and unified baseline for video segmentation. In: Proceedings of the IEEE/CVF Conference on Computer Vision and Pattern Recognition (CVPR), pp. 18847–18857 (2022)
6. Lin, T.Y., Goyal, P., Girshick, R., et al.: Focal loss for dense object detection. In: Proceedings of the IEEE International Conference on Computer Vision (ICCV) (2017)
7. Liu, Y., Shen, C., Yu, C., Wang, J.: Efficient semantic video segmentation with per-frame inference. In: Vedaldi, A., Bischof, H., Brox, T., Frahm, J.-M. (eds.) ECCV 2020. LNCS, vol. 12355, pp. 352–368. Springer, Cham (2020). https://doi.org/10.1007/978-3-030-58607-2_21
8. Miles, R., Yucel, M.K., Manganelli, B., et al.: Mobilevos: real-time video object segmentation contrastive learning meets knowledge distillation. In: Proceedings of the IEEE/CVF Conference on Computer Vision and Pattern Recognition (CVPR), pp. 10480–10490 (2023)
9. Müller, S.G., Hutter, F.: Trivialaugment: tuning-free yet state-of-the-art data augmentation. In: Proceedings of the IEEE/CVF International Conference on Computer Vision (ICCV), pp. 774–782 (2021)
10. Psychogyios, D., Colleoni, E., Van Amsterdam, B., et al.: Sar-rarp50: segmentation of surgical instrumentation and action recognition on robot-assisted radical prostatectomy challenge (2024)

11. Ravi, N., Gabeur, V., Hu, Y.T., et al.: Sam 2: segment anything in images and videos. arXiv preprint arXiv:2408.00714 (2024)
12. Ronneberger, O., Fischer, P., Brox, T.: U-Net: convolutional networks for biomedical image segmentation. In: Navab, N., Hornegger, J., Wells, W.M., Frangi, A.F. (eds.) MICCAI 2015. LNCS, vol. 9351, pp. 234–241. Springer, Cham (2015). https://doi.org/10.1007/978-3-319-24574-4_28
13. Ross, T., Reinke, A., Full, P.M., et al.: Robust medical instrument segmentation challenge 2019 (2020)
14. Sudre, C.H., Li, W., Vercauteren, T., Ourselin, S., Jorge Cardoso, M.: Generalised dice overlap as a deep learning loss function for highly unbalanced segmentations. In: Cardoso, M.J., et al. (eds.) DLMIA/ML-CDS -2017. LNCS, vol. 10553, pp. 240–248. Springer, Cham (2017). https://doi.org/10.1007/978-3-319-67558-9_28
15. Tan, M., Le, Q.: EfficientNet: rethinking model scaling for convolutional neural networks. In: Chaudhuri, K., Salakhutdinov, R. (eds.) Proceedings of the 36th International Conference on Machine Learning. Proceedings of Machine Learning Research, vol. 97, pp. 6105–6114. PMLR (2019)
16. Tu, Z., Talebi, H., Zhang, H., et al.: Maxvit: multi-axis vision transformer. In: ECCV (2022)
17. Wang, Y., Lipson, L., Deng, J., et al.: SEA-RAFt: simple, efficient, accurate RAFT for optical flow. In: Leonardis, A., Ricci, E., Roth, S., et al. (eds.) Computer Vision – ECCV 2024, pp. 36–54. Springer (2025)
18. Zia, A., Bhattacharyya, K., Liu, X., et al.: Surgical tool classification and localization: results and methods from the MICCAI 2022 surgtoolloc challenge (2023)

Author Index

N. Akash et al. (Eds.): EMERGE 2025 Workshops, LNCS 16534, pp. 145–146, 2026.
https://doi.org/10.1007/978-3-032-24182-5

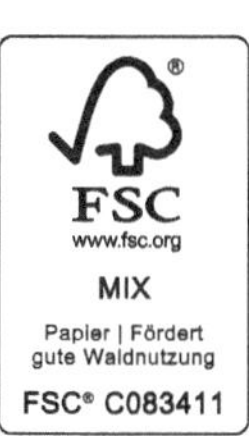

Zeitfracht Medien GmbH
Ferdinand-Jühlke-Straße 7
99095 Erfurt, Deutschland
produktsicherheit@kolibri360.de